Meditate with
Mandalas

D.E. Boone

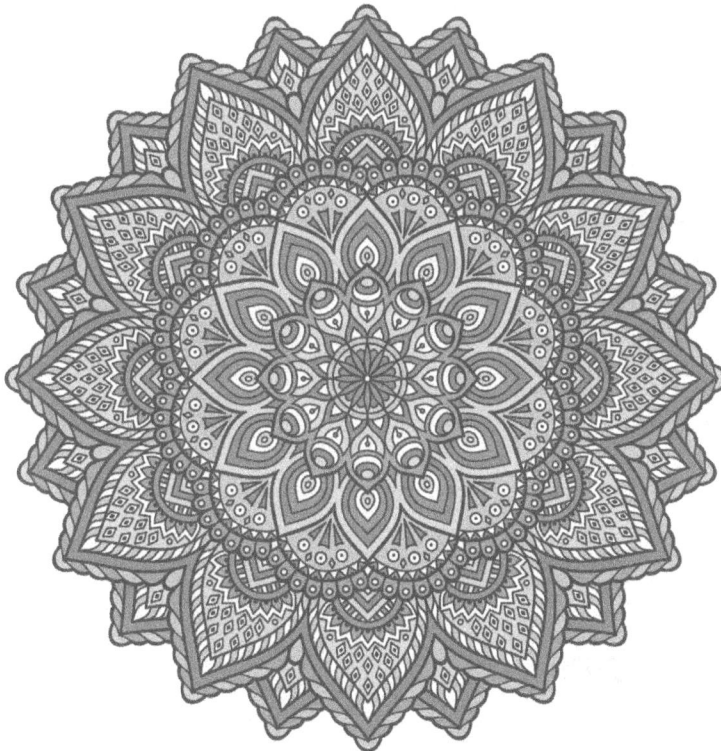

FOR▶▶WARD
MOTION PUBLISHING

Forward Motion Publishing LLC
Jamaica, NY 11432

Forward Motion Publishing is an indie publisher focused on compiling
helpful, fun and inspiring books for adults.

ISBN 978-0692600740

FOR▶▶WARD
MOTION PUBLISHING

What exactly is a Mandala?

Mandala's are spiritual symbols that represent the Universe. They are historically used as an aid to meditation and as an way to focus and calm the mind. A Mandala is a simple geometric shape that has no beginning or end. Within its circular shape, the mandala has the power to promote relaxation.

Why Adult Coloring Books?

With the pressures of modern life taking a firmer grip on our daily lives, we need to experience inner peace more now than ever. Coloring is a stress-free activity that relaxes your brain and calms your fears. It allows your mind to get the rest it needs.

Coloring is a meditative, free-time activity you can schedule, making it perfect for retraining your brain to respond less harshly to stress.

Even more, coloring requires the two hemispheres of your brain to communicate, and the activity itself improves your fine motor skills and vision. Coloring books, much like crossword puzzles, are very therapeutic.

Why Meditate with Mandalas?

Mandalas are used to promote healing and other positive states of being. The healing powers of Mandala's comes from its design. The mandala is a circular matrix with a center point—a point from which all things are possible. From this sacred center comes forth infinite possibilities and unlimited potential.

When you use your mandala coloring pages, you're expressing your desires for healing and wellness. Amazing as it sounds, by simply coloring mandalas, you can accomplish the following:

Relax your mind
Balance your body, your mind, and your spirit
Make a spiritual connection
Expand your creativity
Improves your focus
Encourage your self-expression
Just have fun, alone or with your friends

Coloring Mandalas

Mandalas represent wholeness and connections to the universe.

Within the pages of this publication you will find over fifty hypnotic mandalas that pulse with life and energy.

Mandalas are designed to relax you. So go ahead and get centered.

Simply by mandala coloring, you may find yourself calm.

Instructions

Just add color. In any way you like.

Don't feel like you have to stay between the lines, unless you want too.

Breath deeply and give yourself permission to experienced the calm that comes from coloring Mandalas.

Listen to relaxing music while you color.

Meditate with the Mandalas.

I have so much chaos in my life, it's become normal. You become used to it. You have to just relax, calm down, take a deep breath and try to see how you can make things work rather than complain about how they're wrong.

–Tom Welling

Tips

Each of these relaxing mandalas is perfect for coloring with markers, watercolors, colored pencils, gel pens, or crayons.

If you are using markers, you might want to put a piece of scrap paper between the pages you want to color.

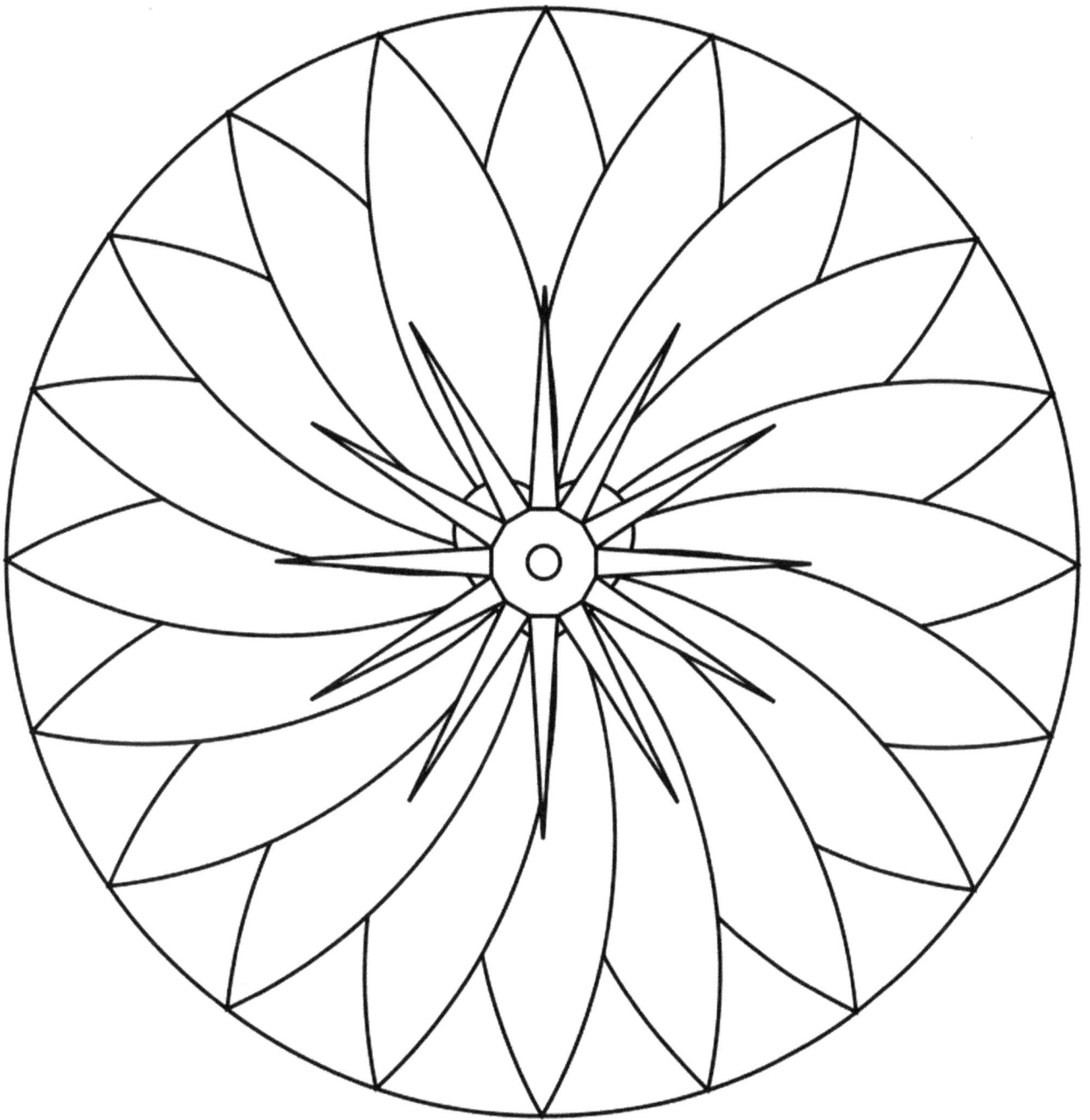

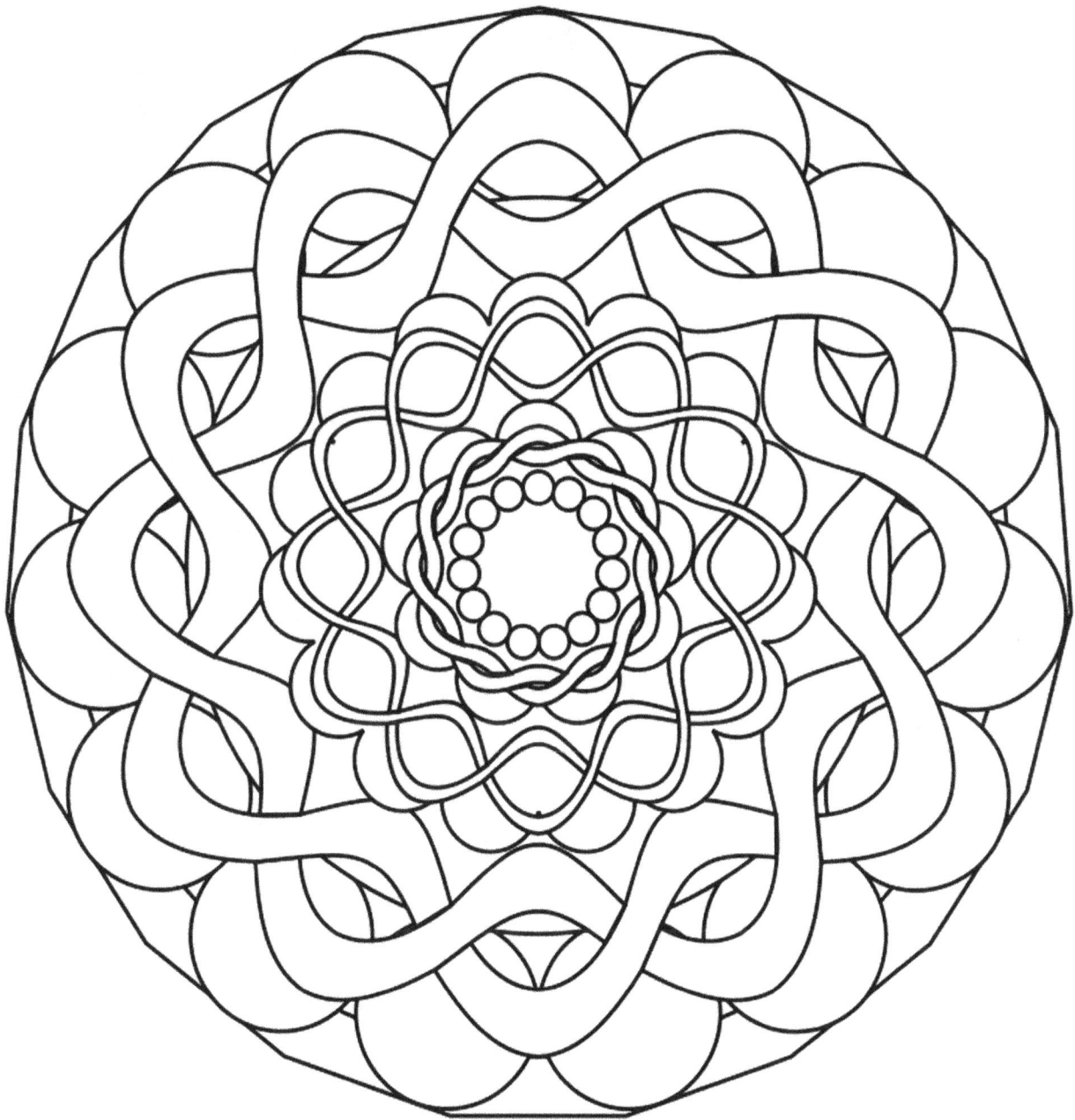

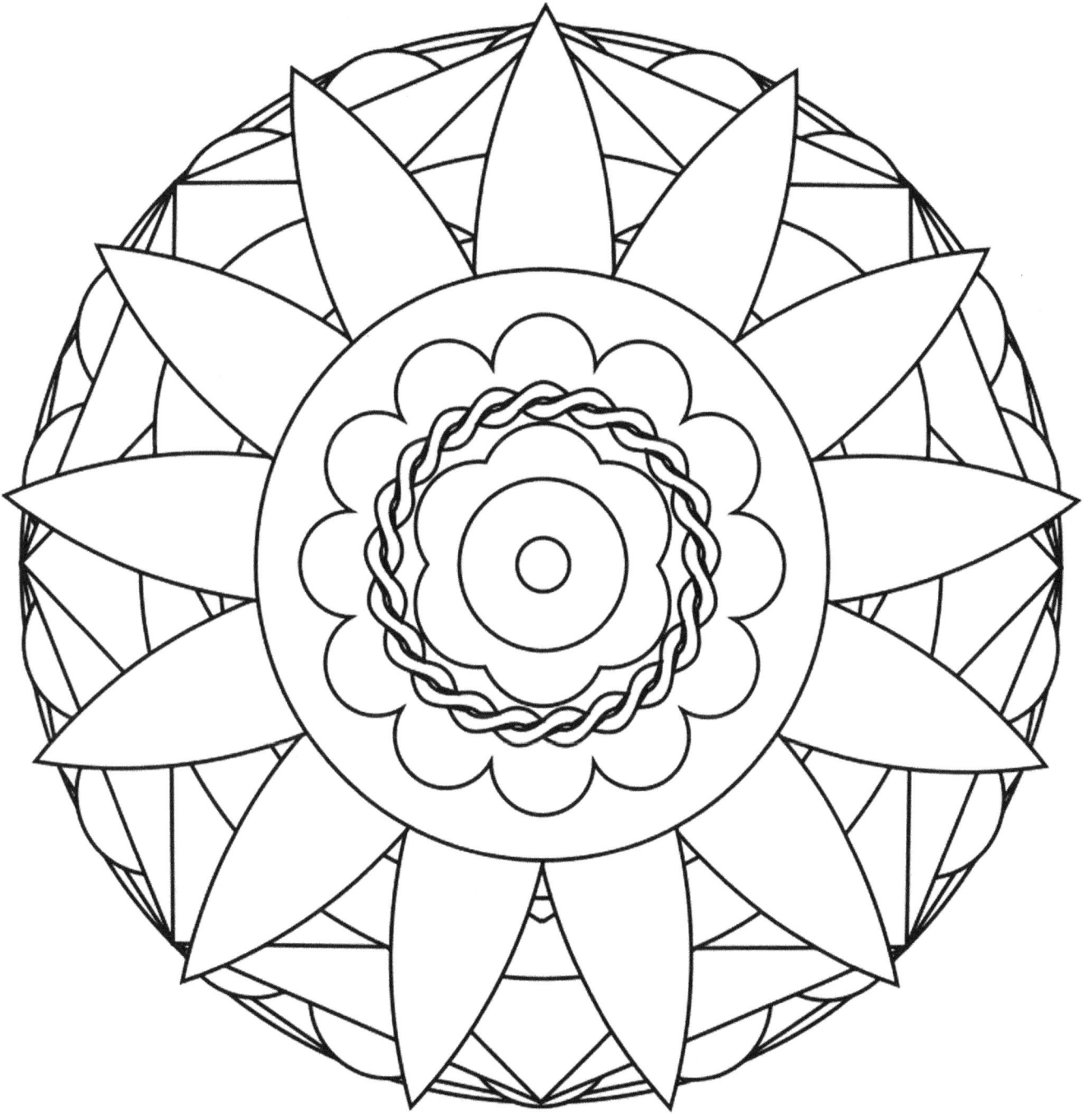

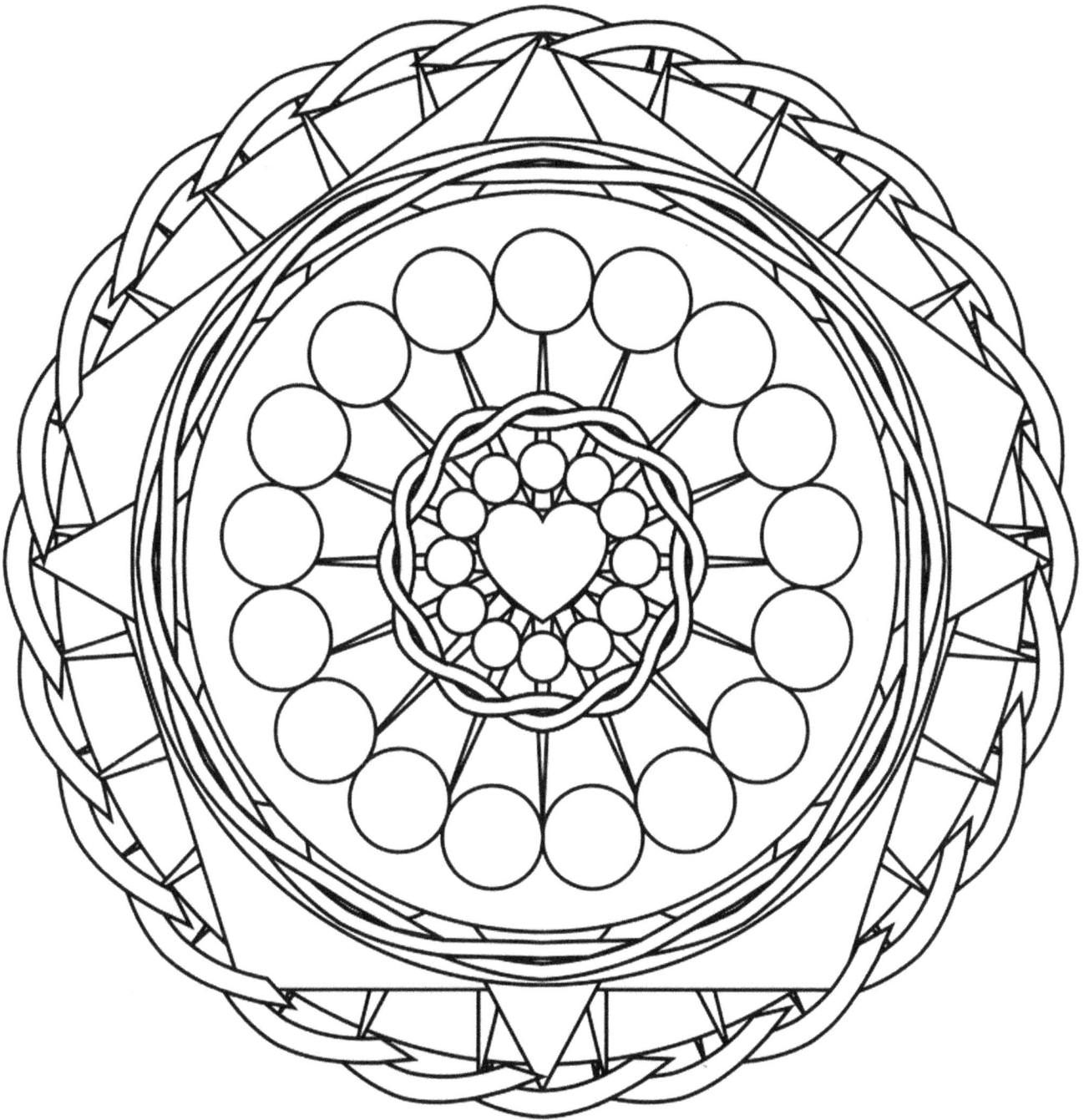

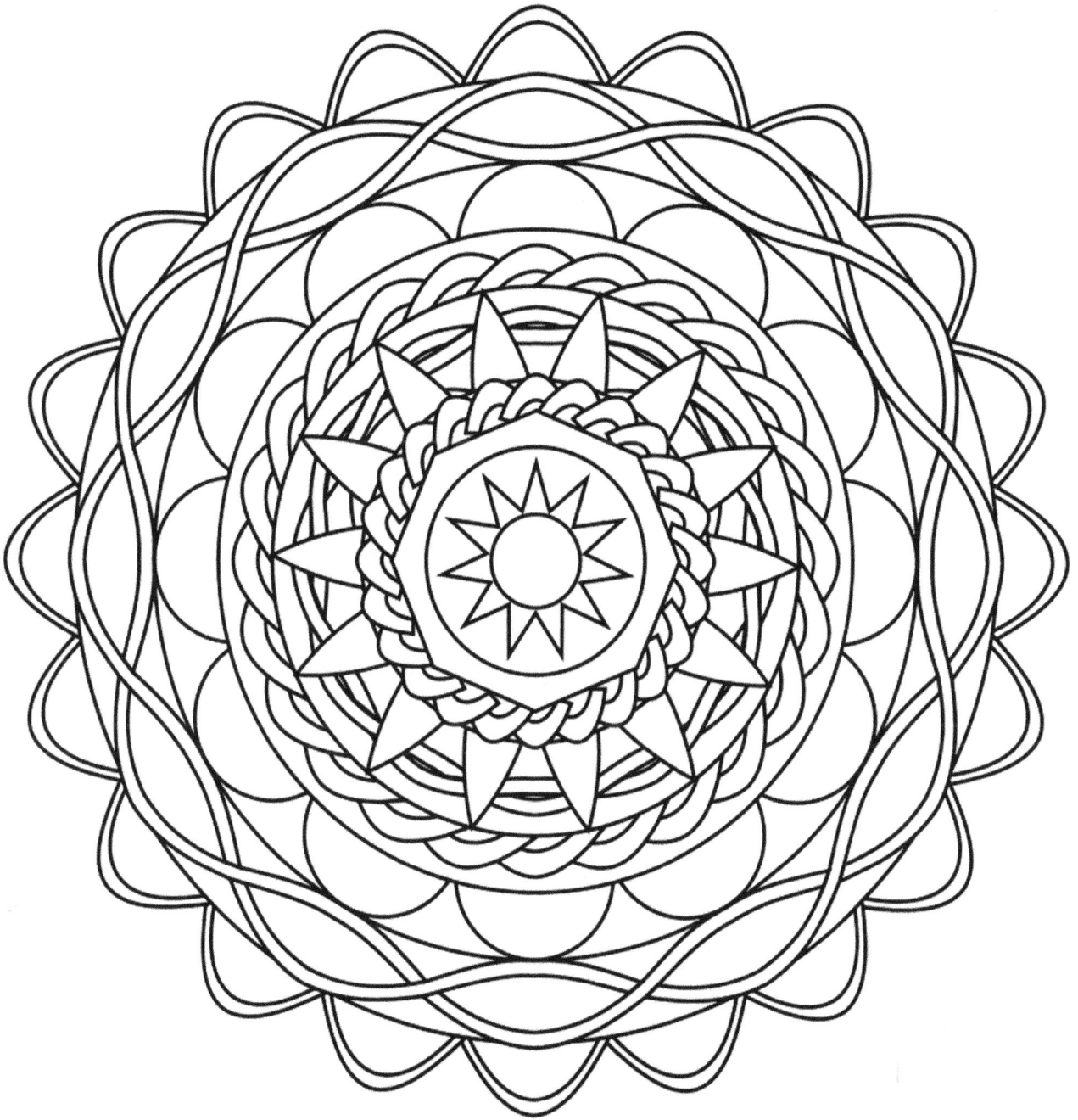

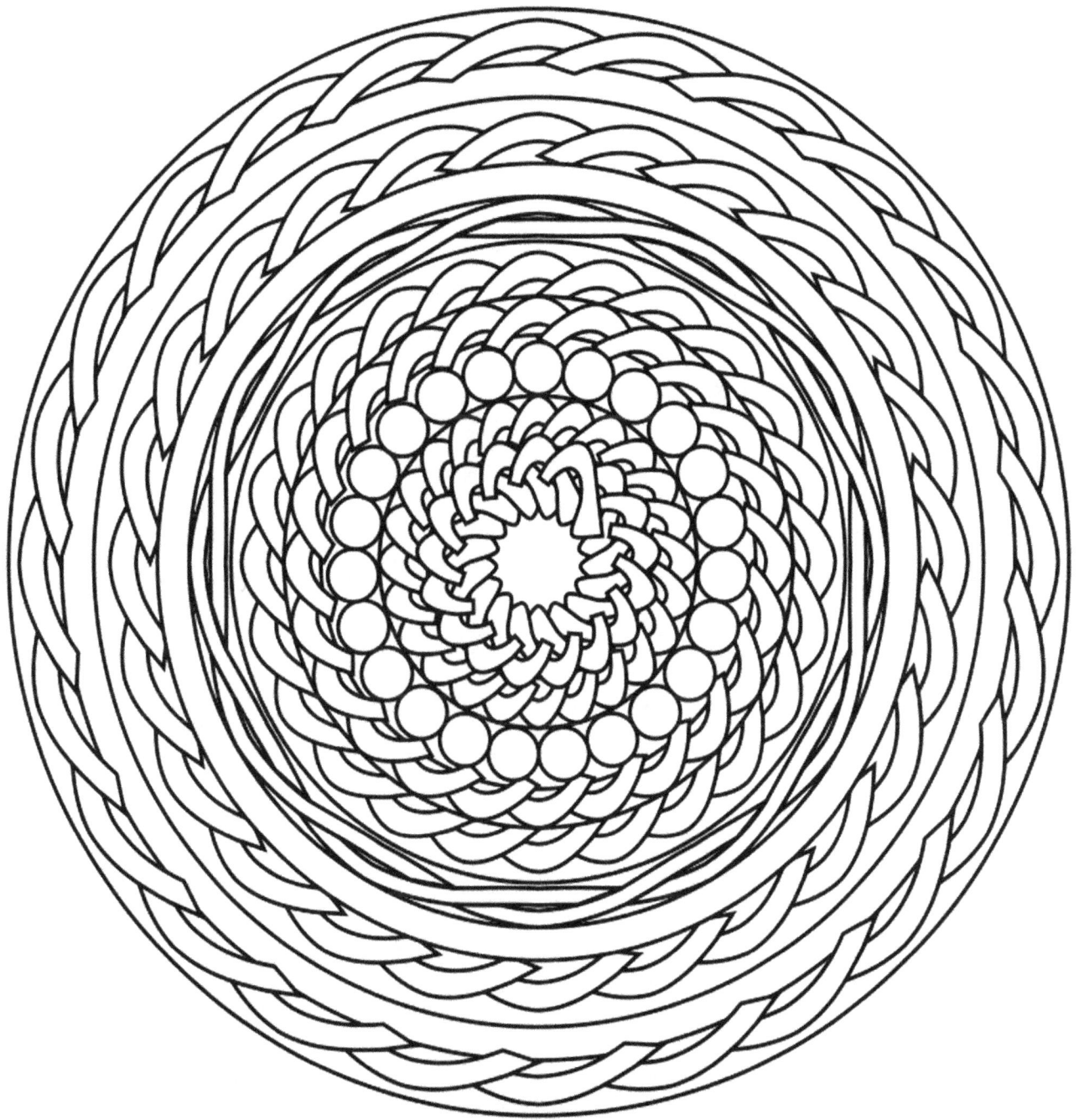

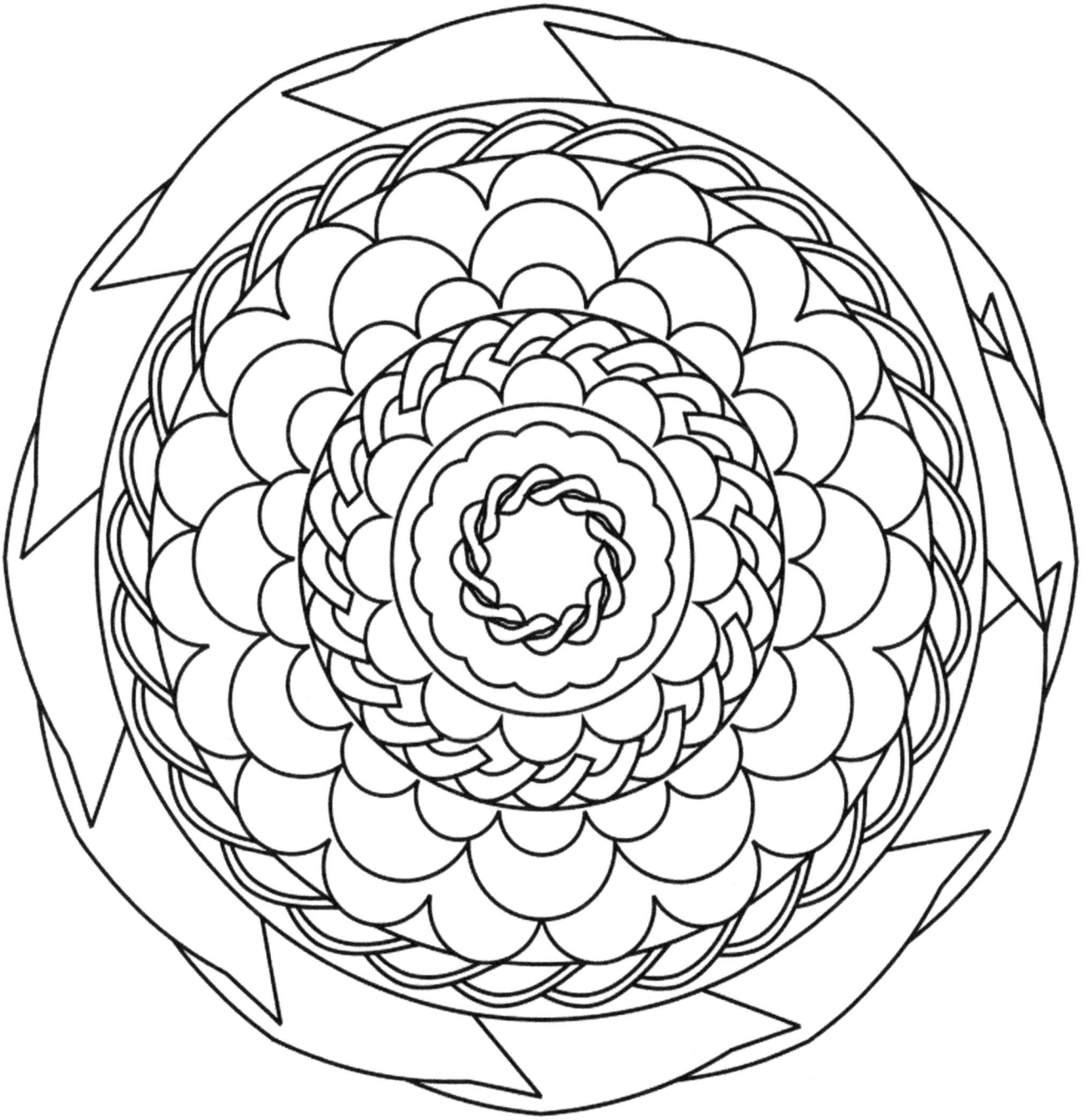

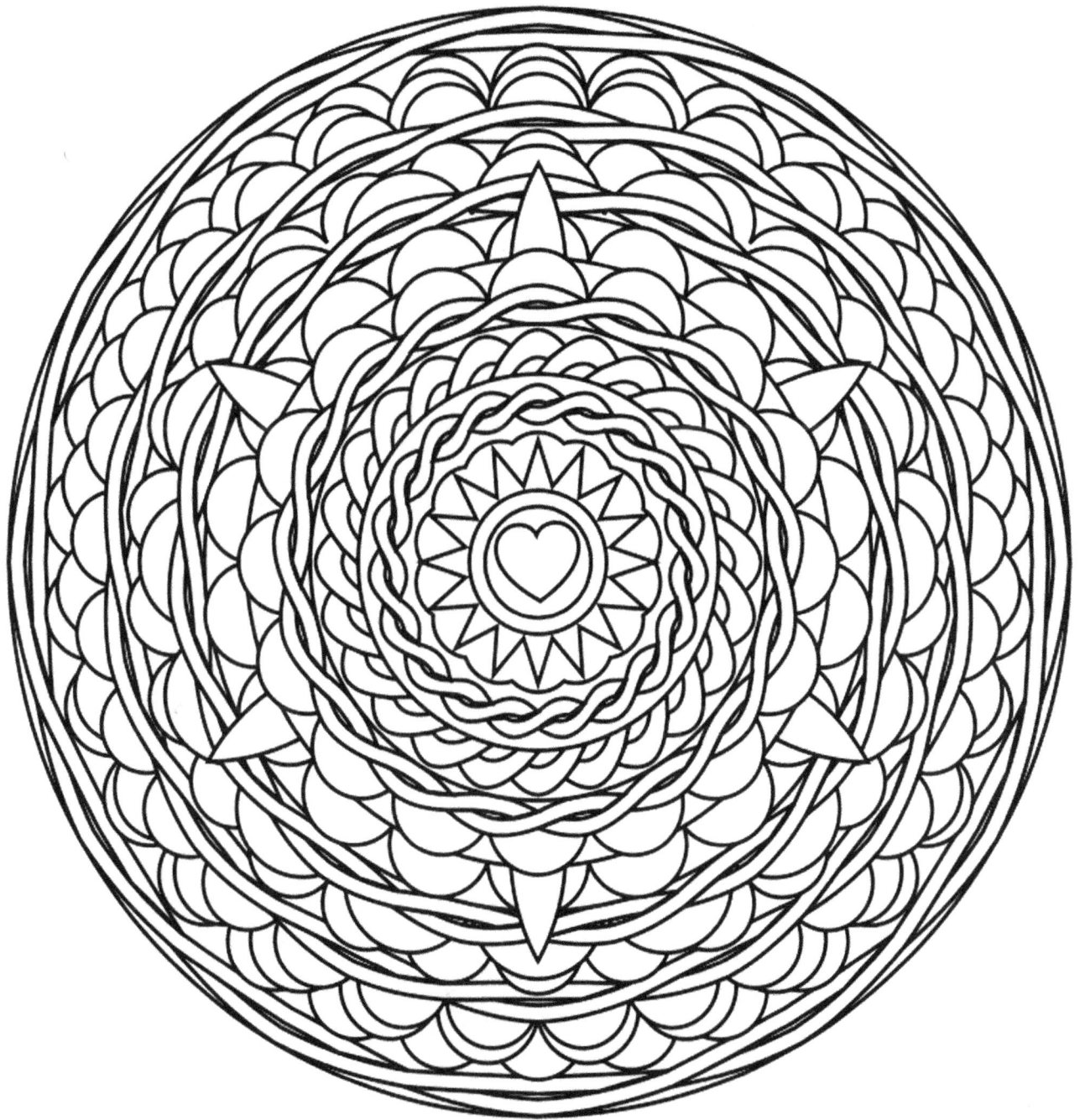

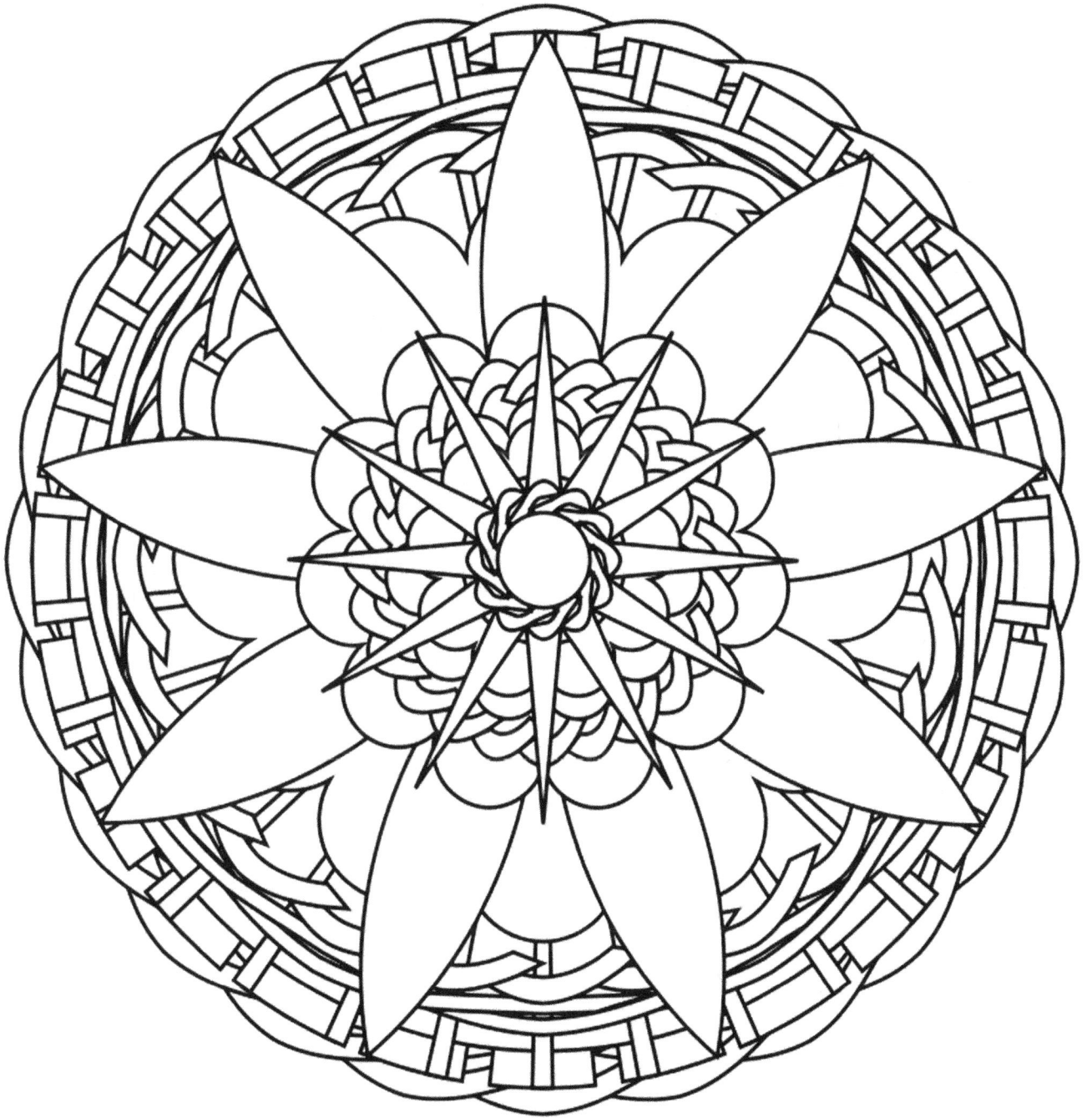

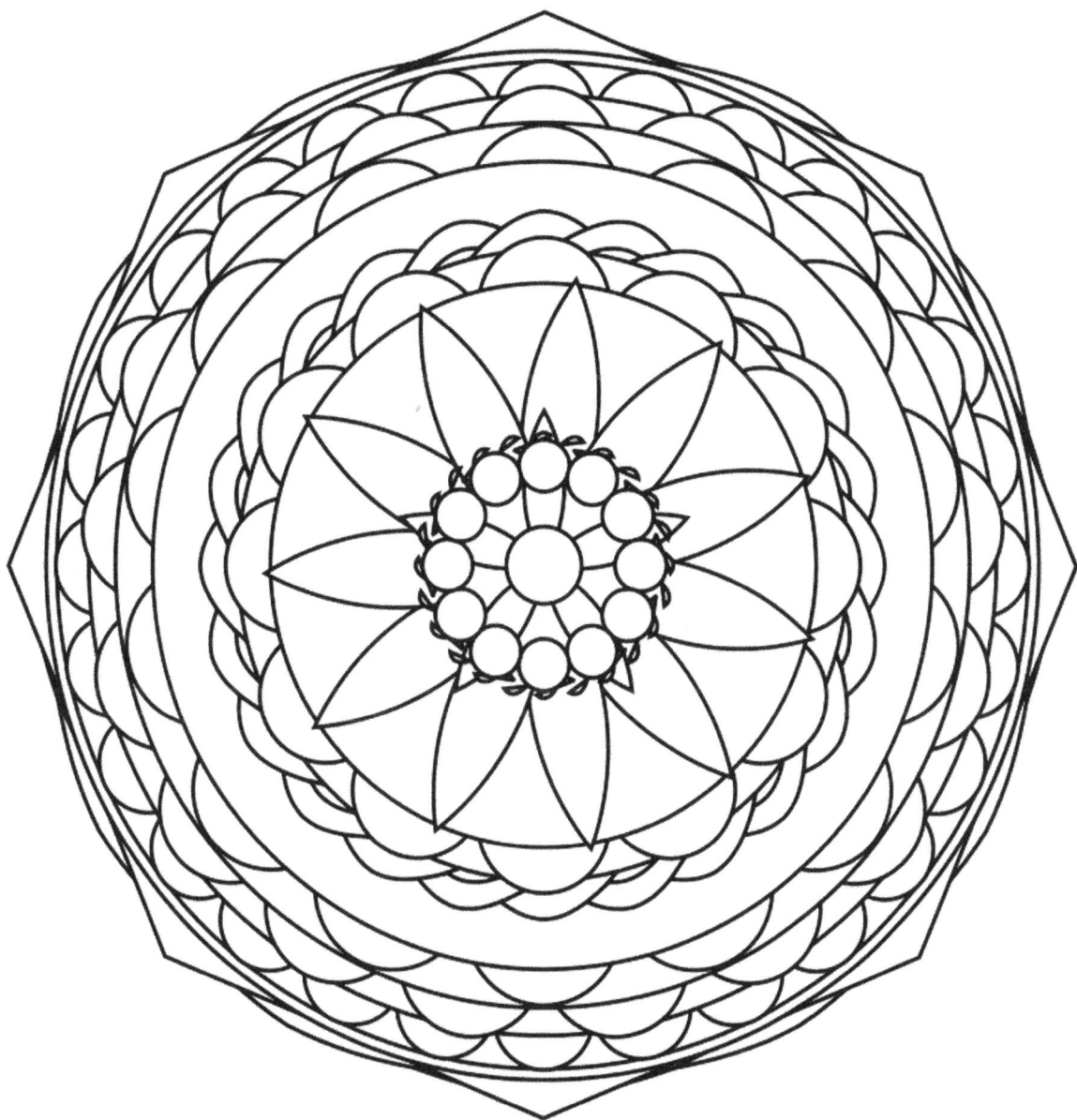

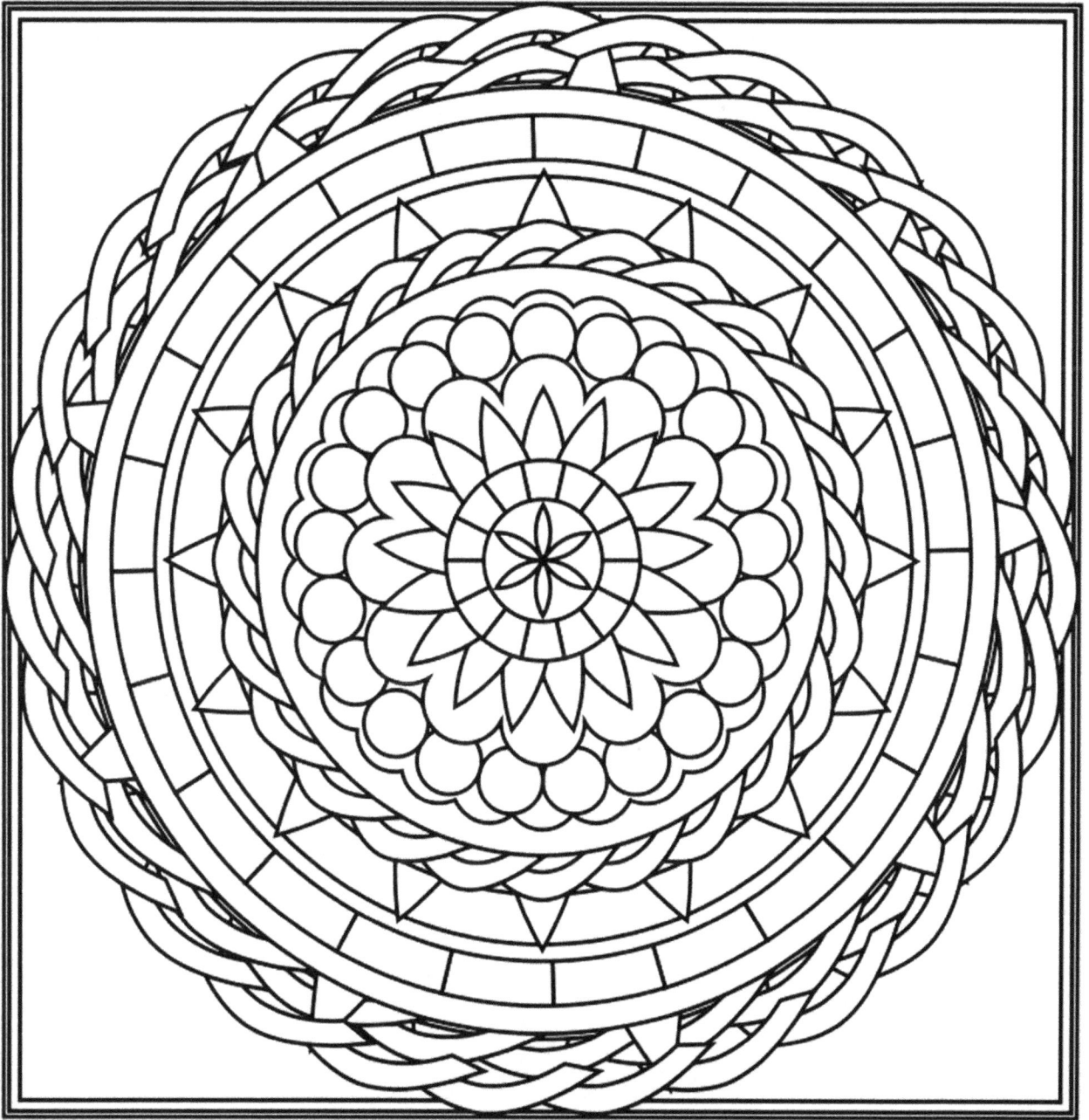

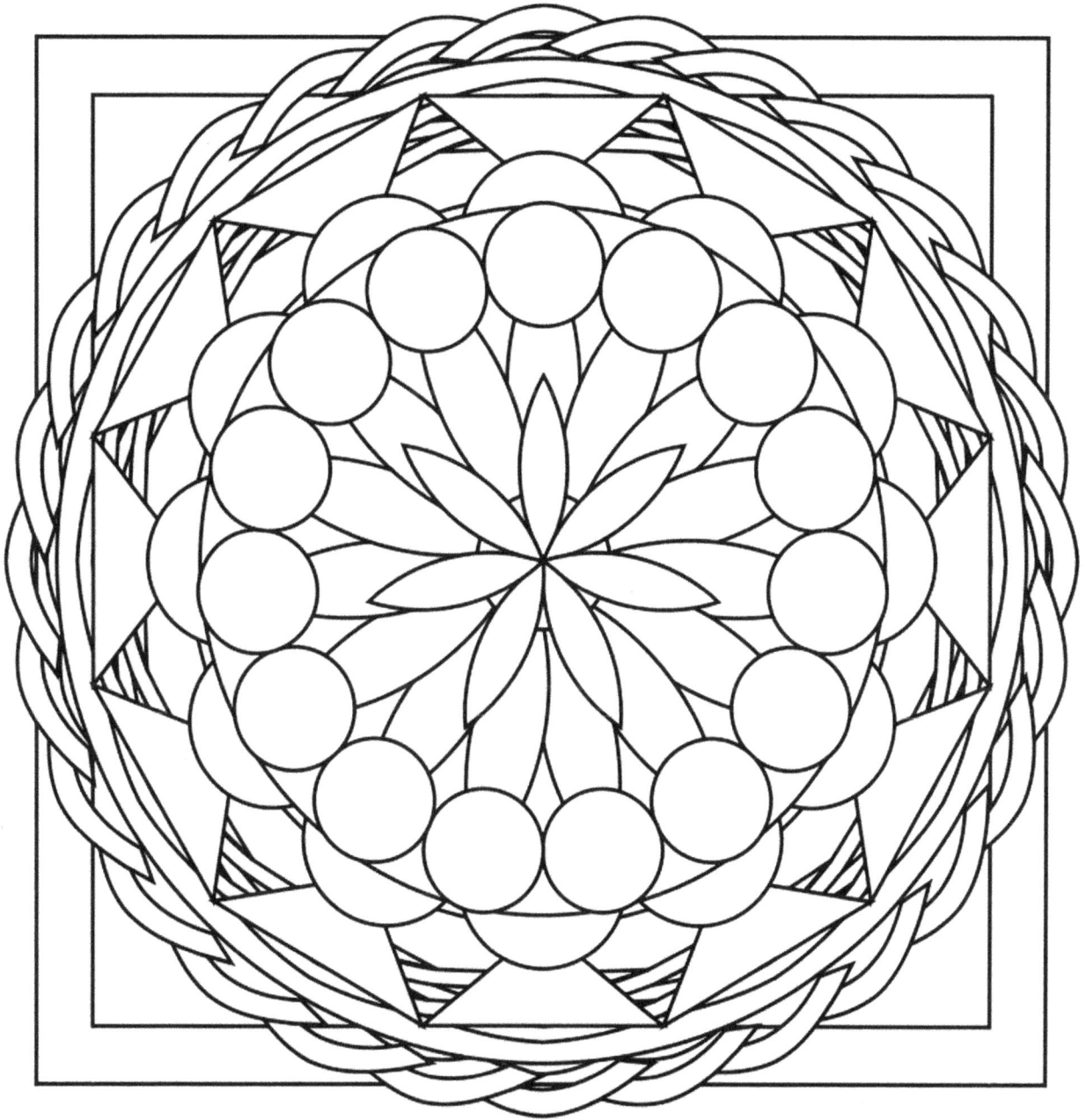

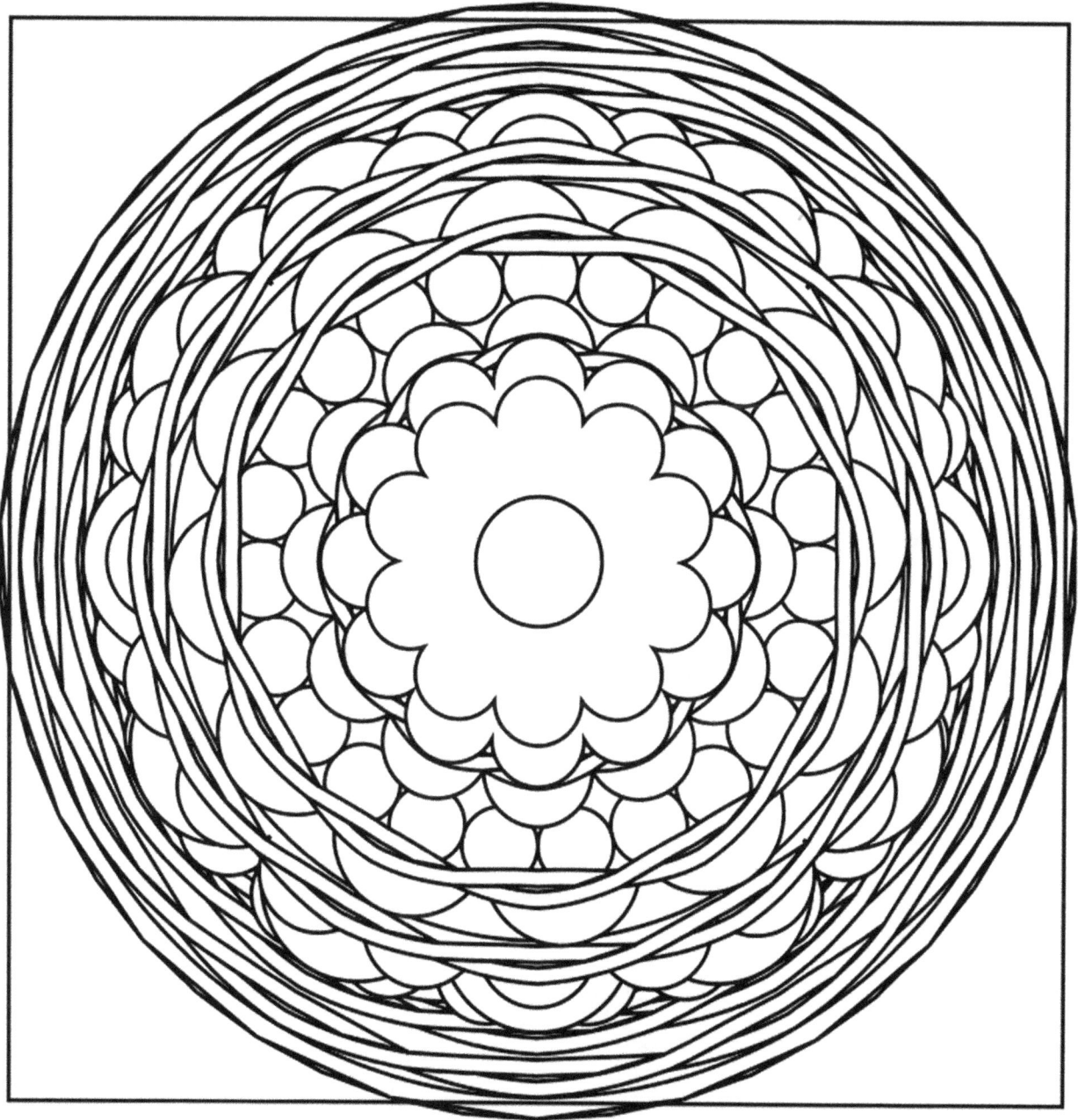

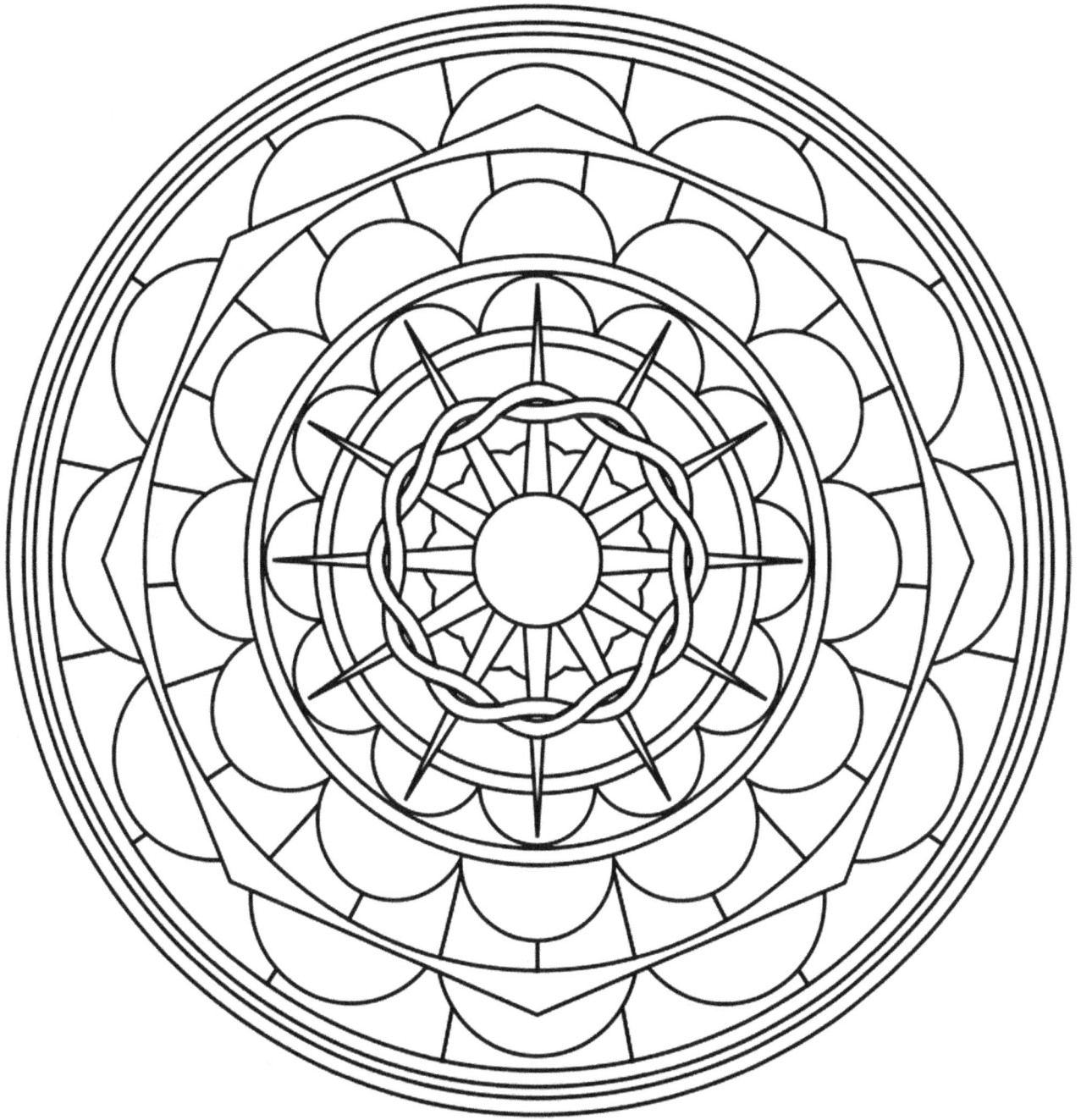

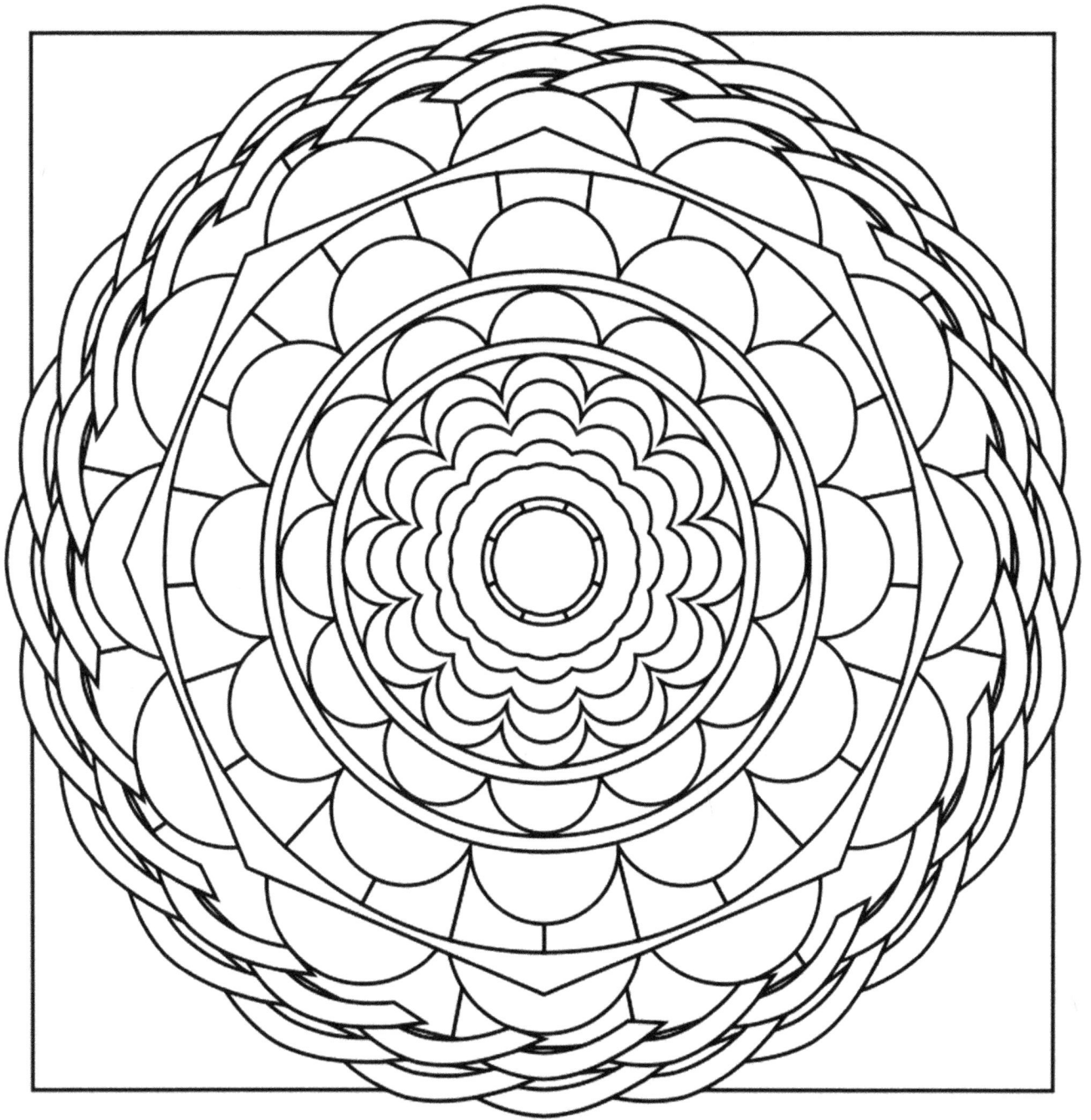

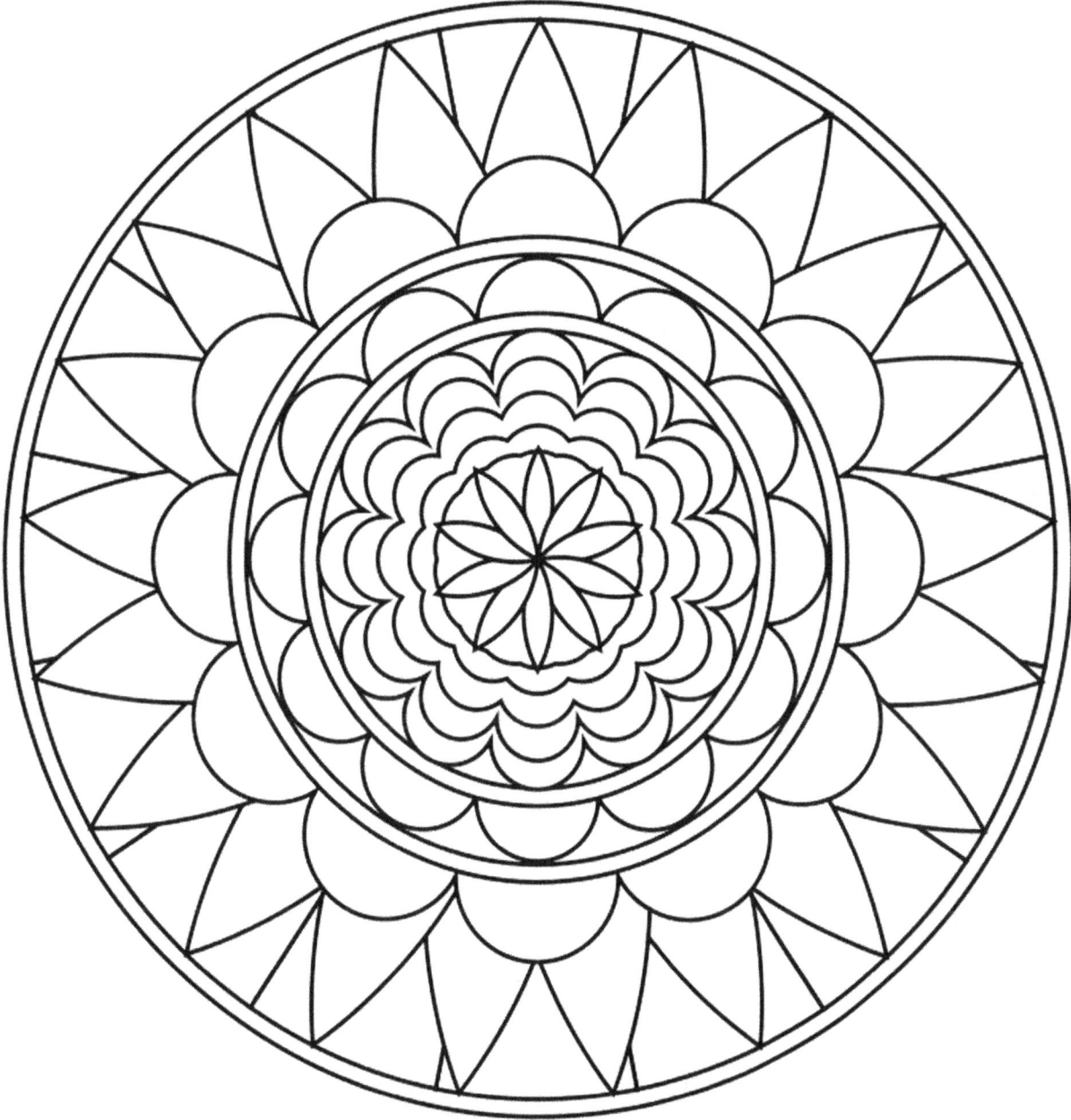

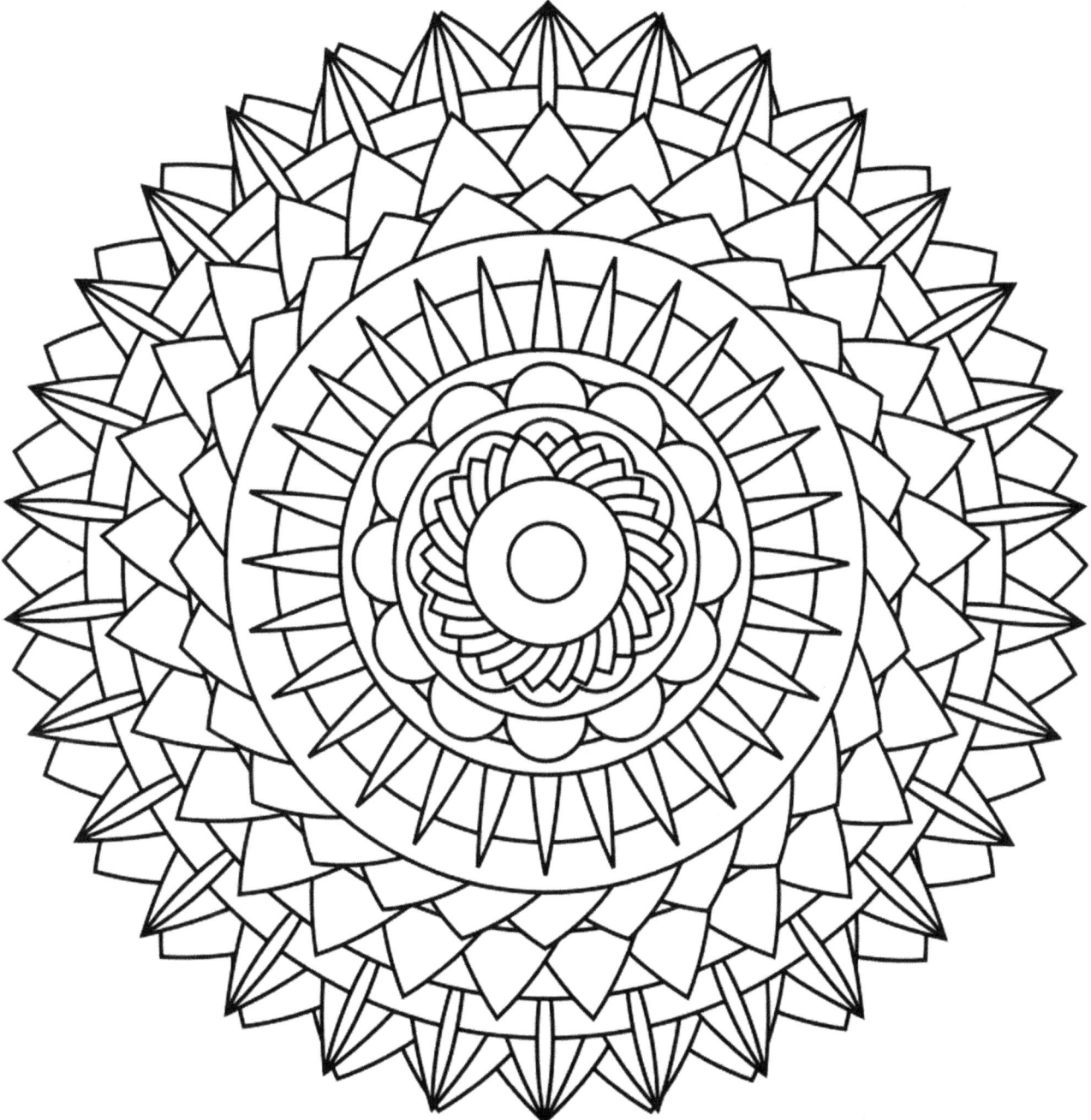

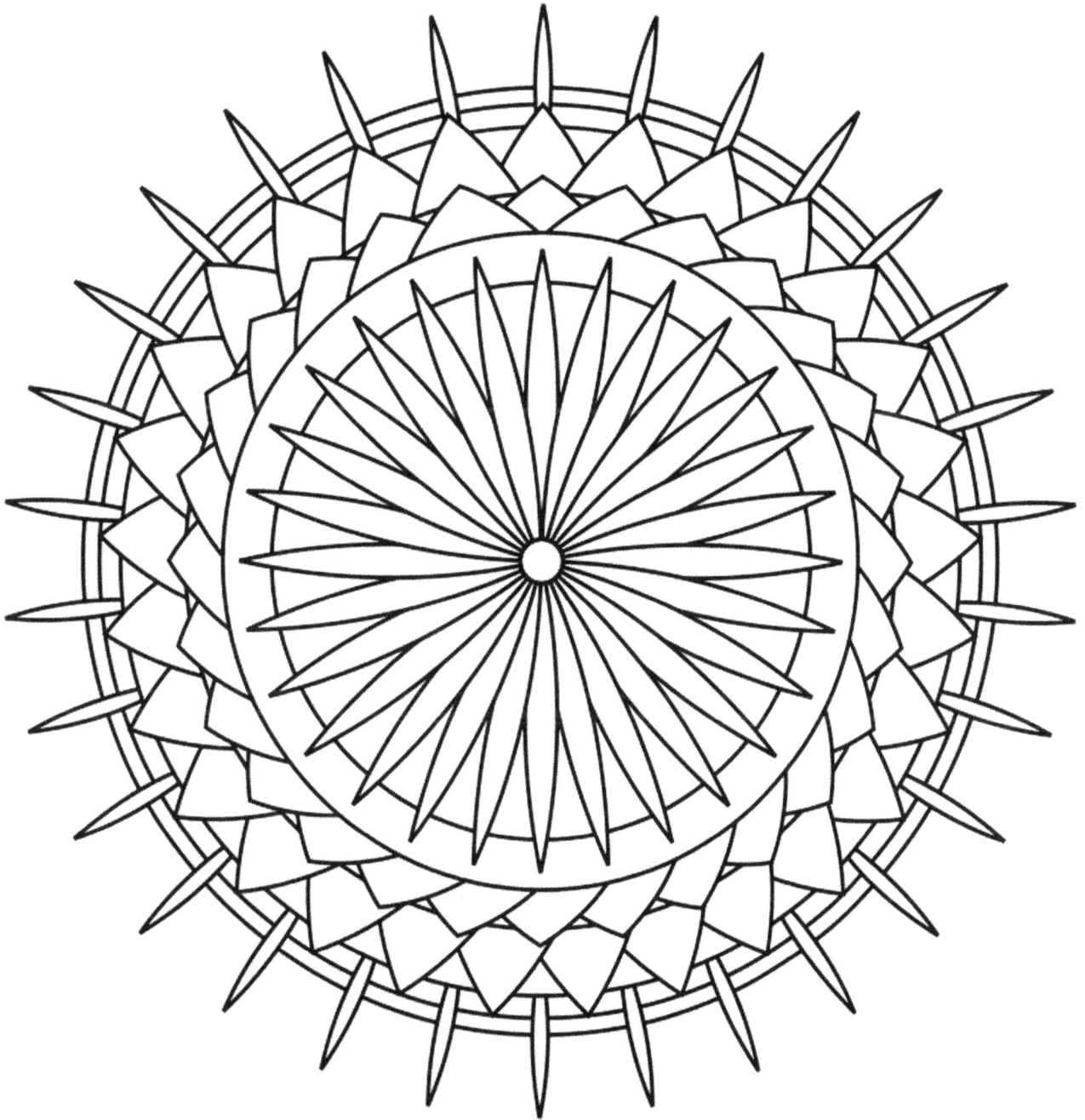

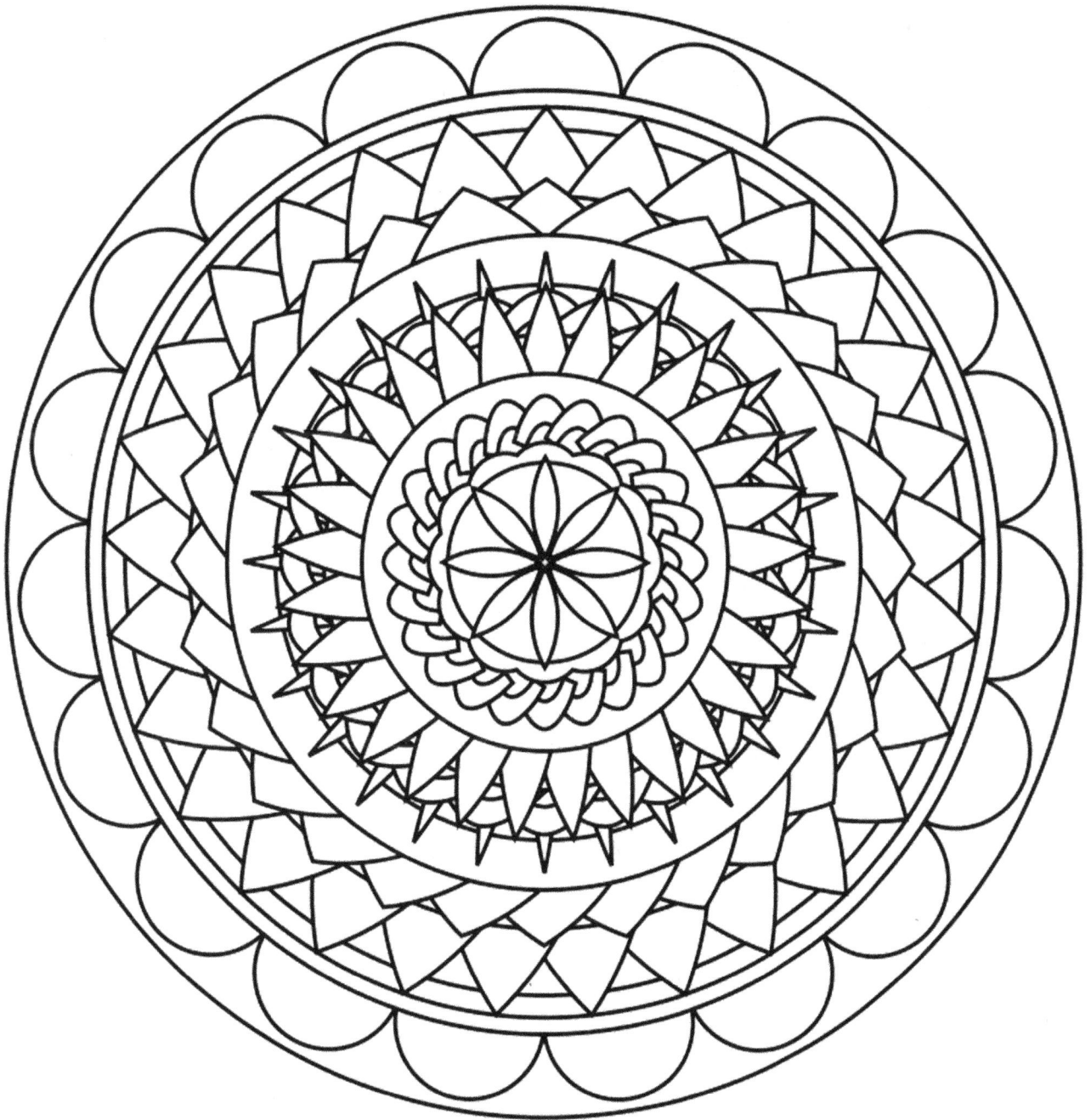

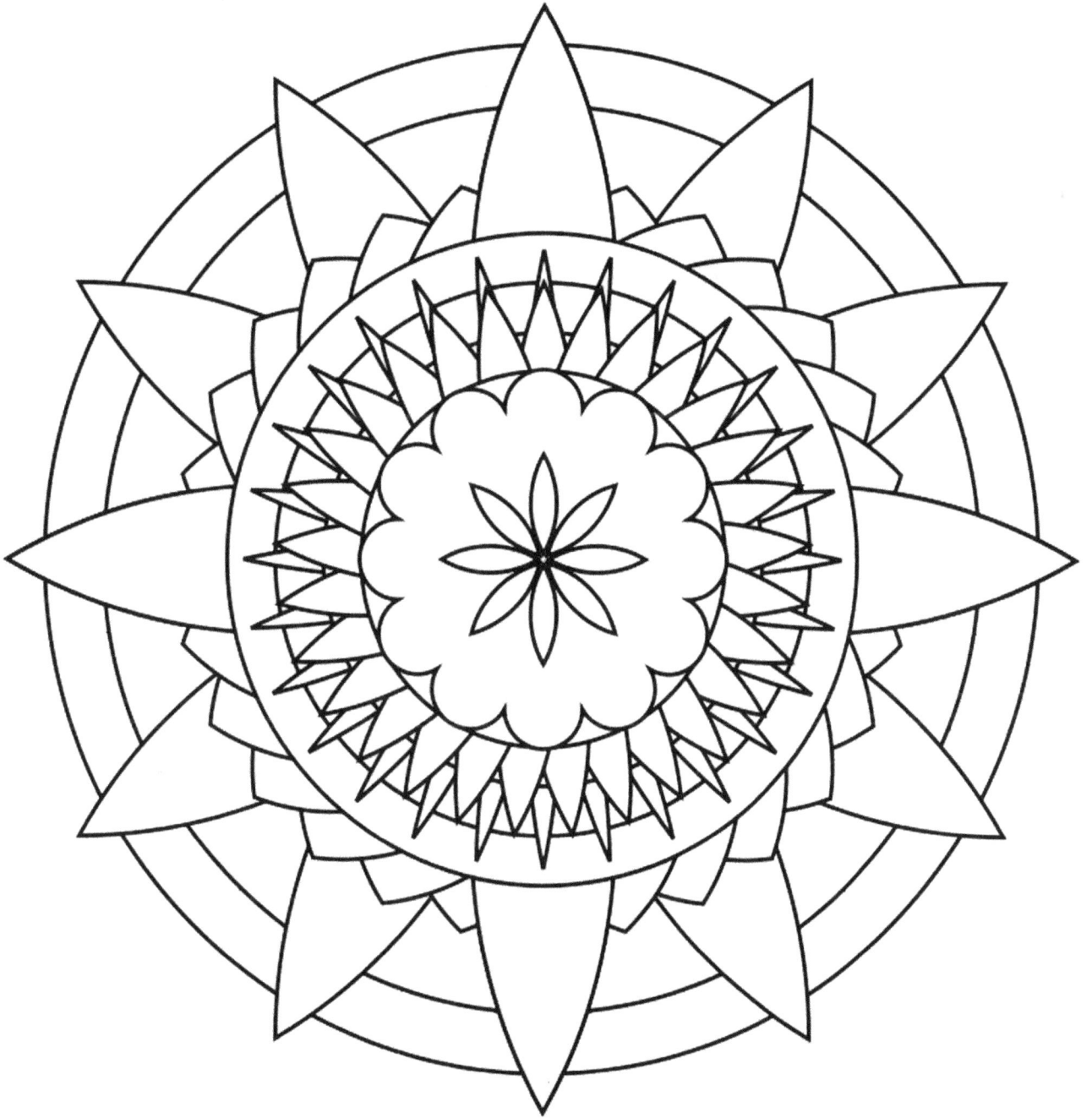

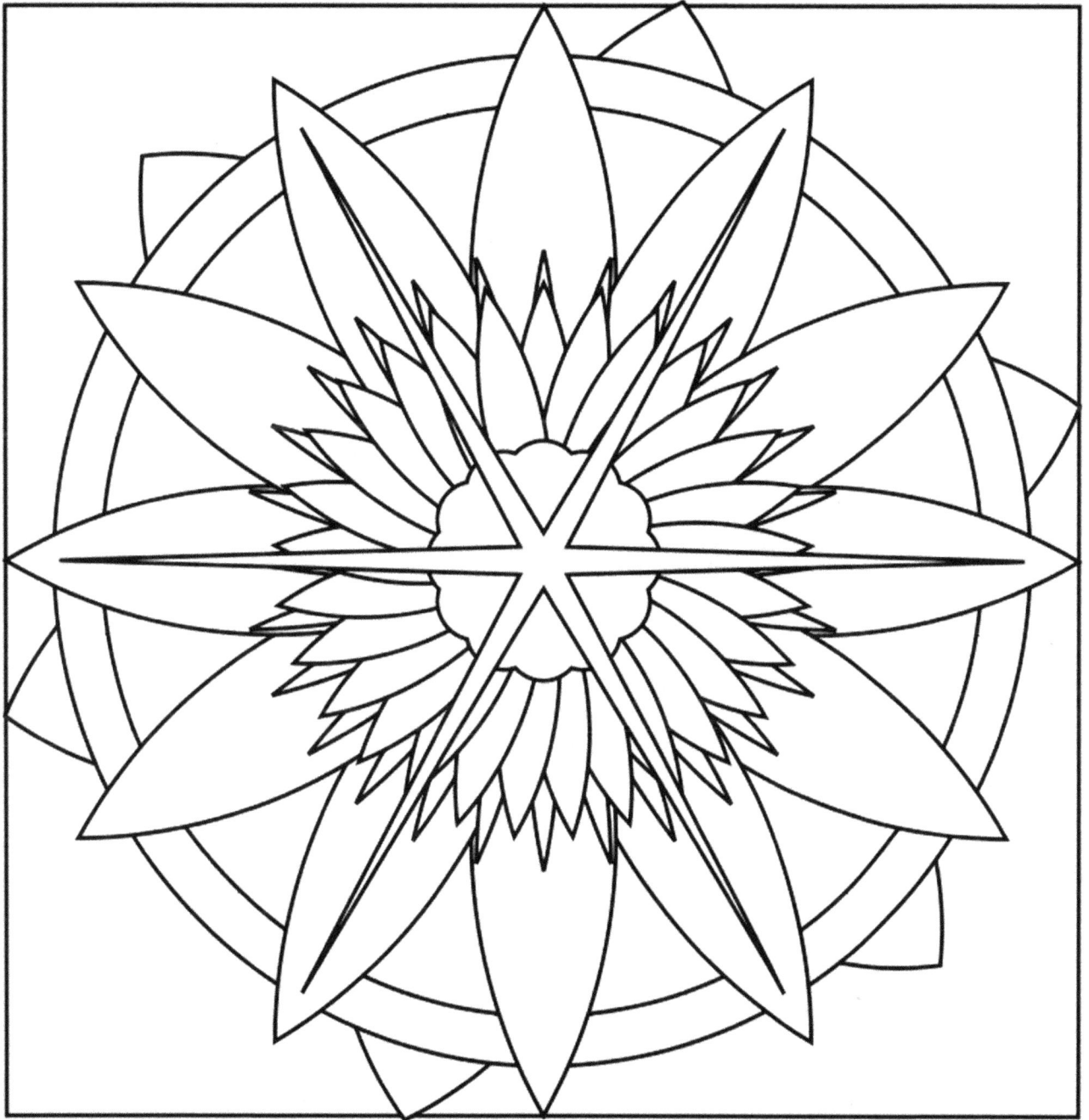

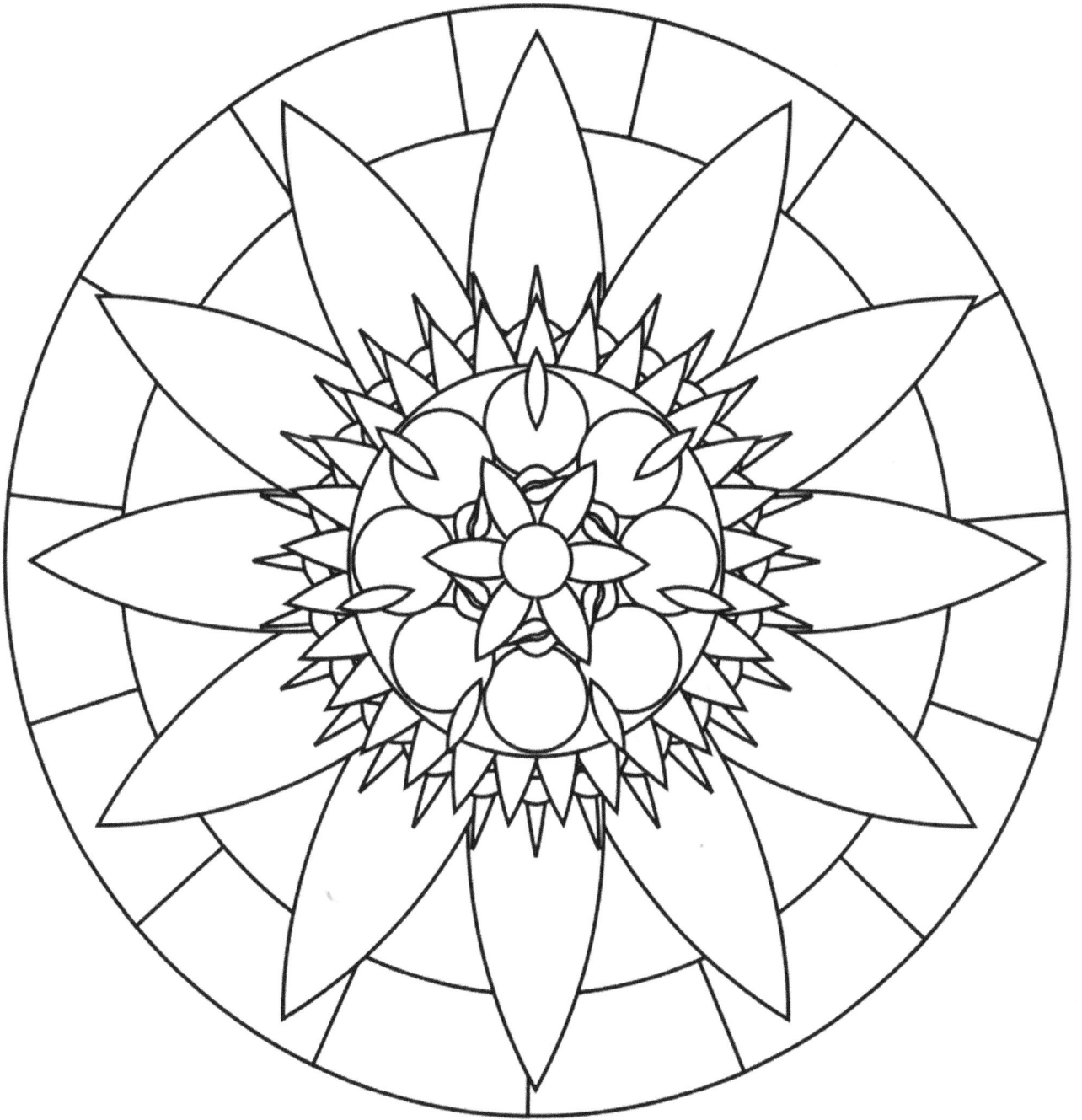

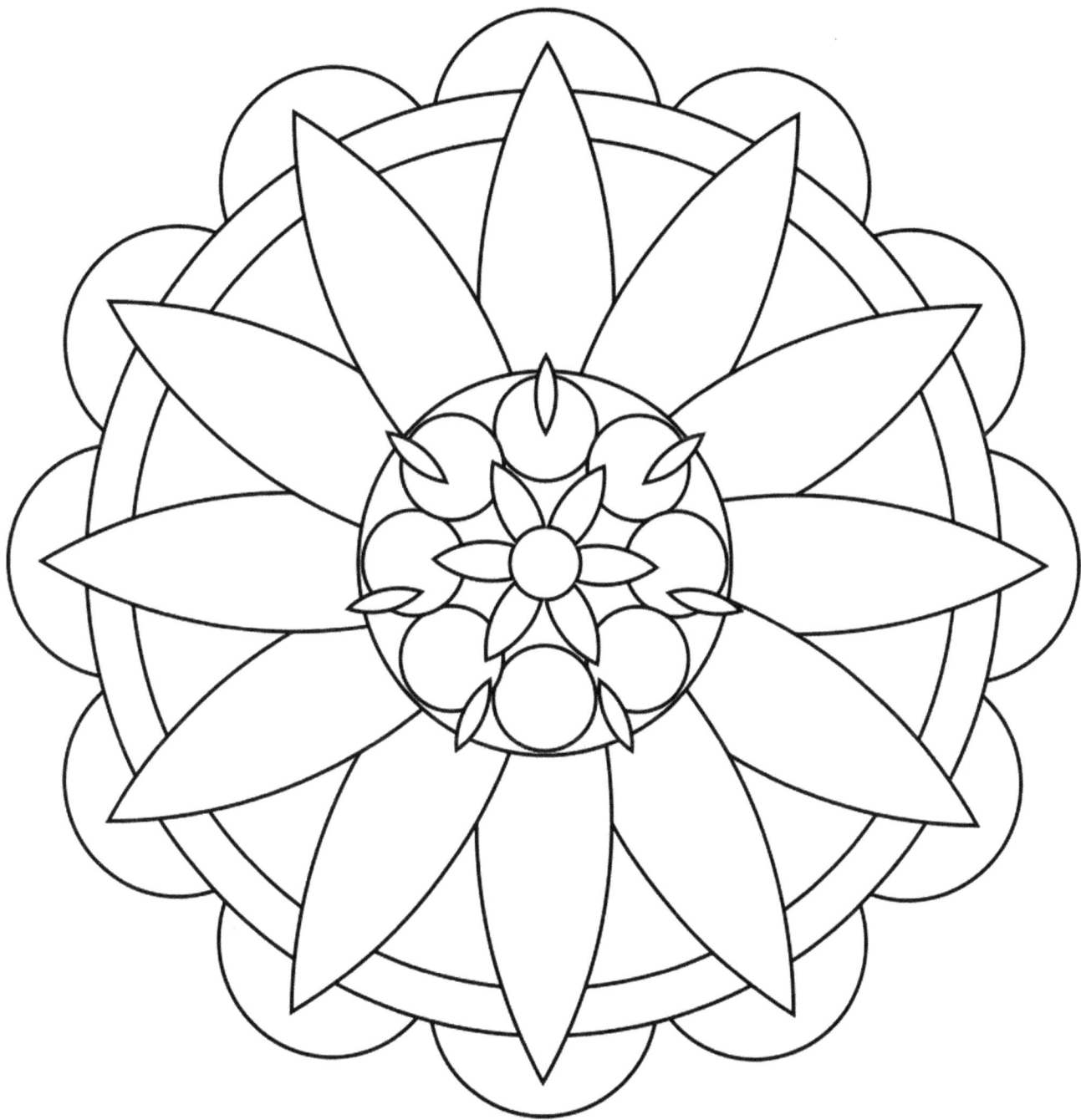

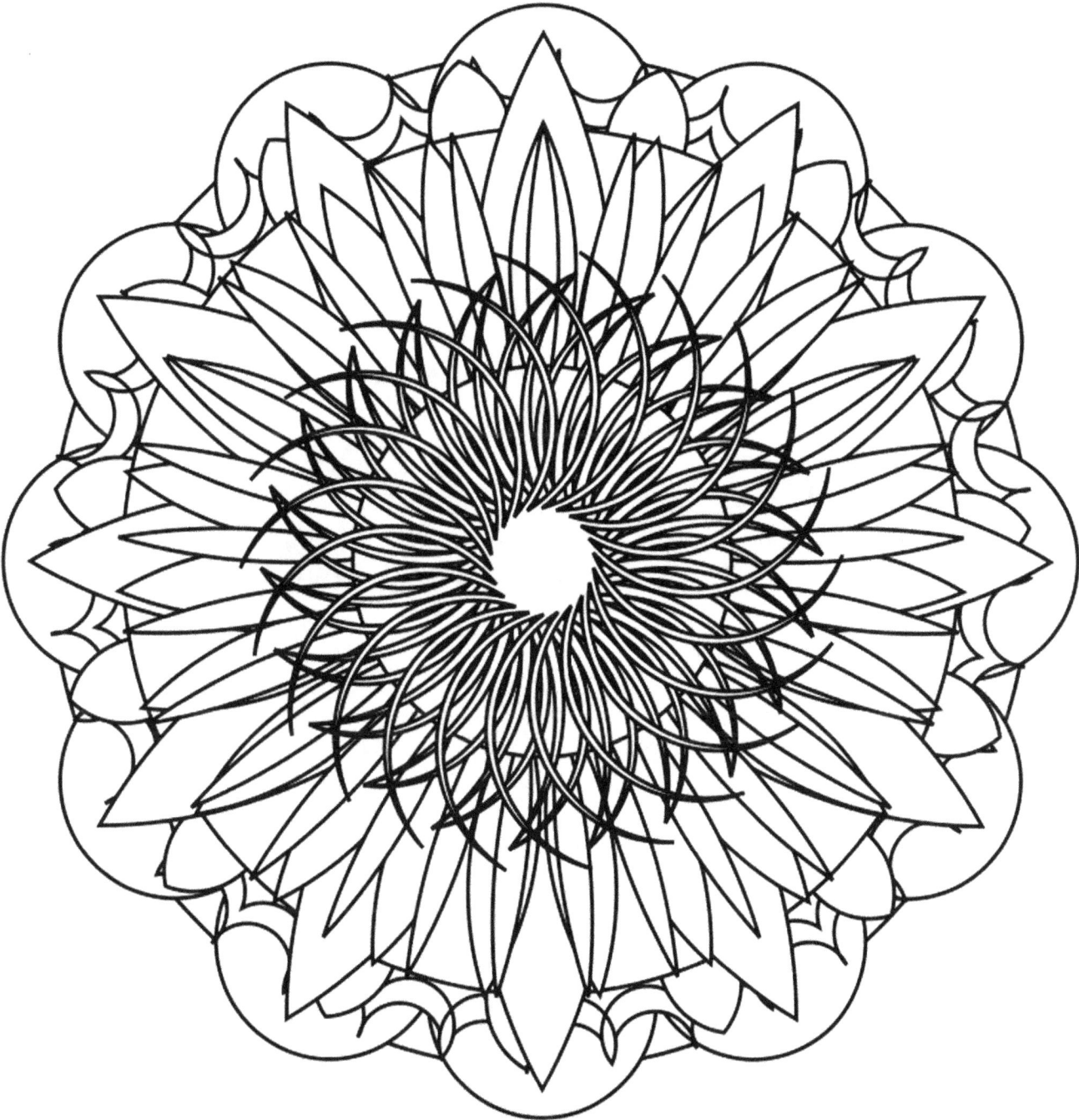

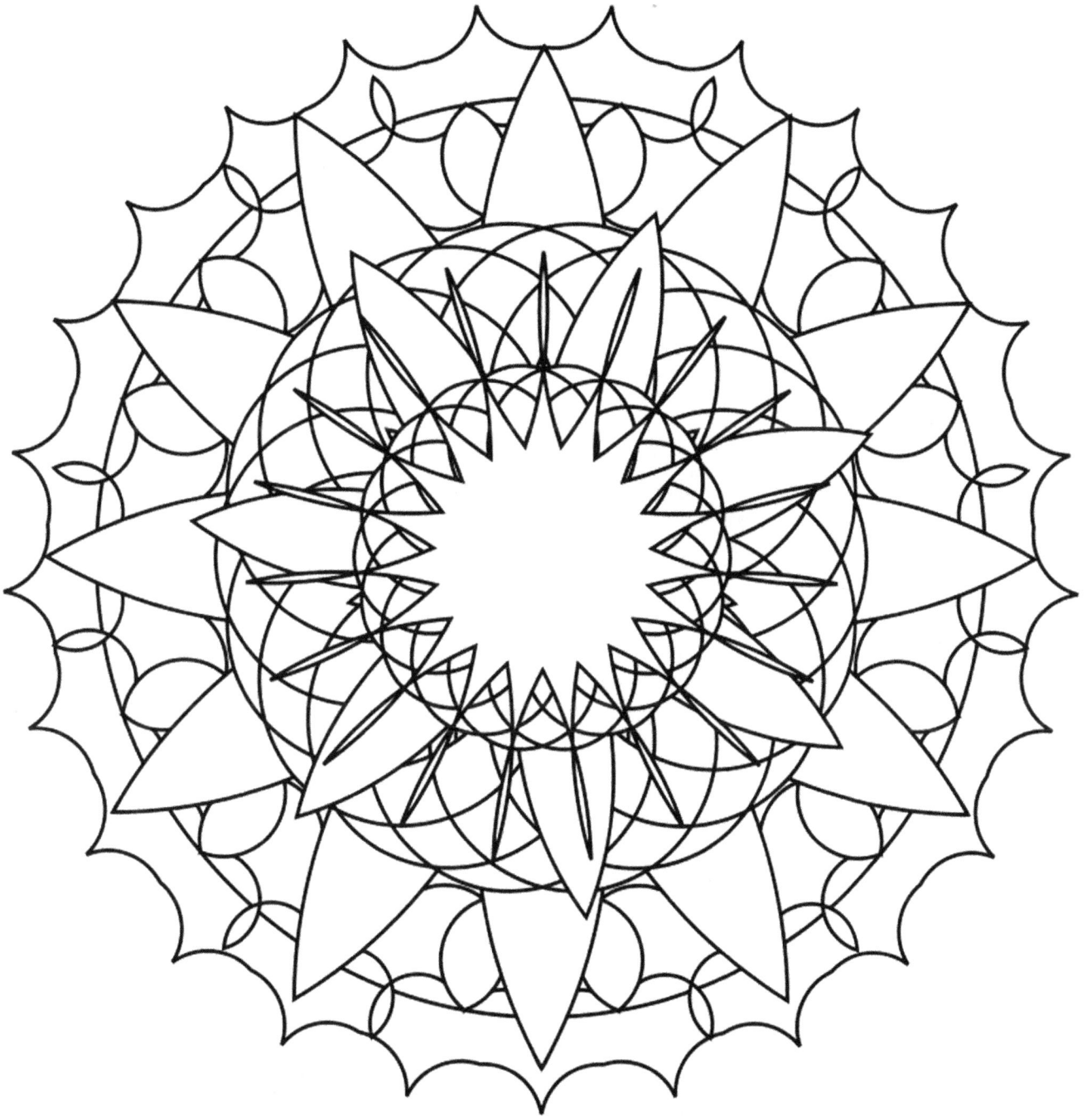

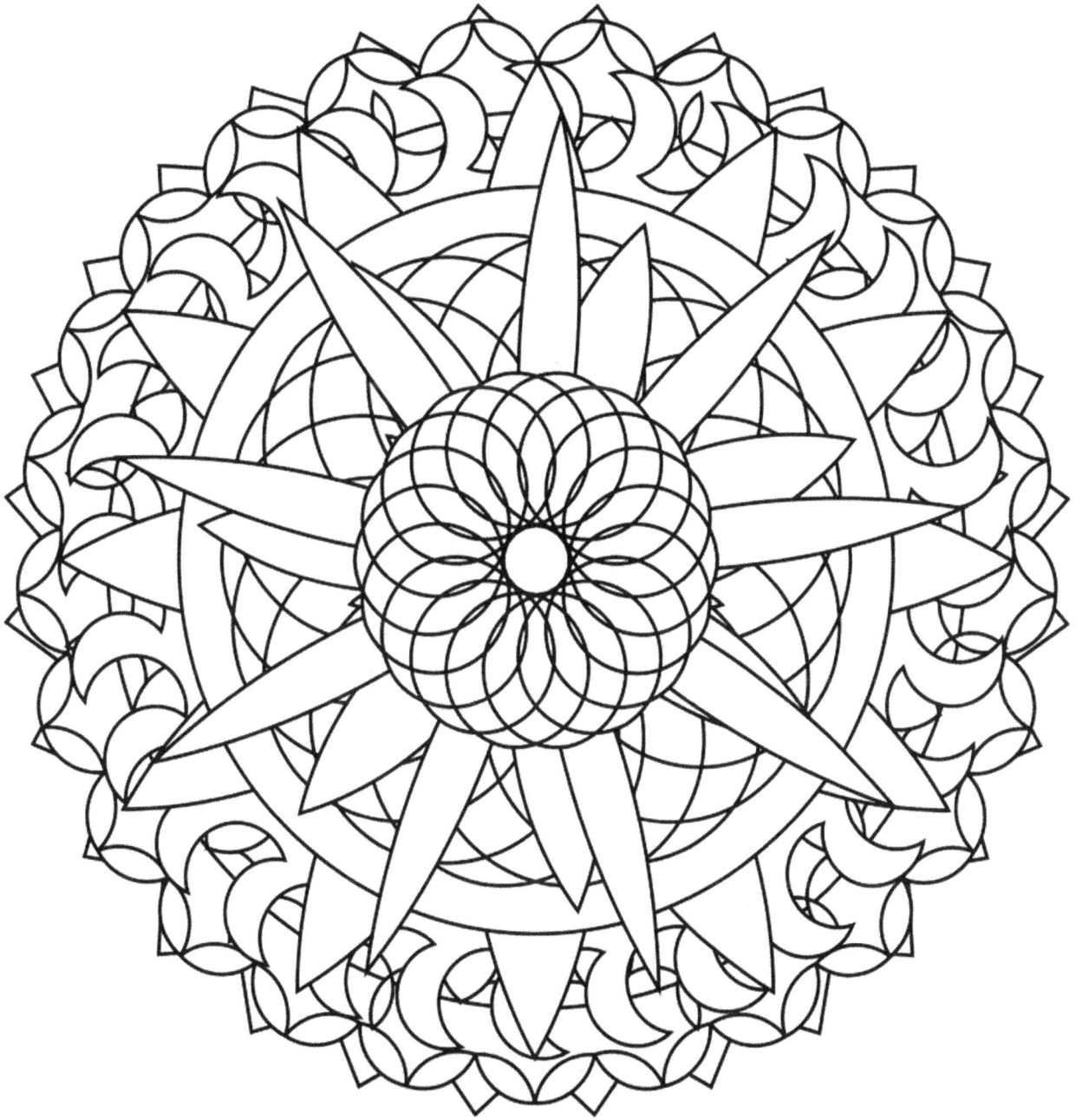

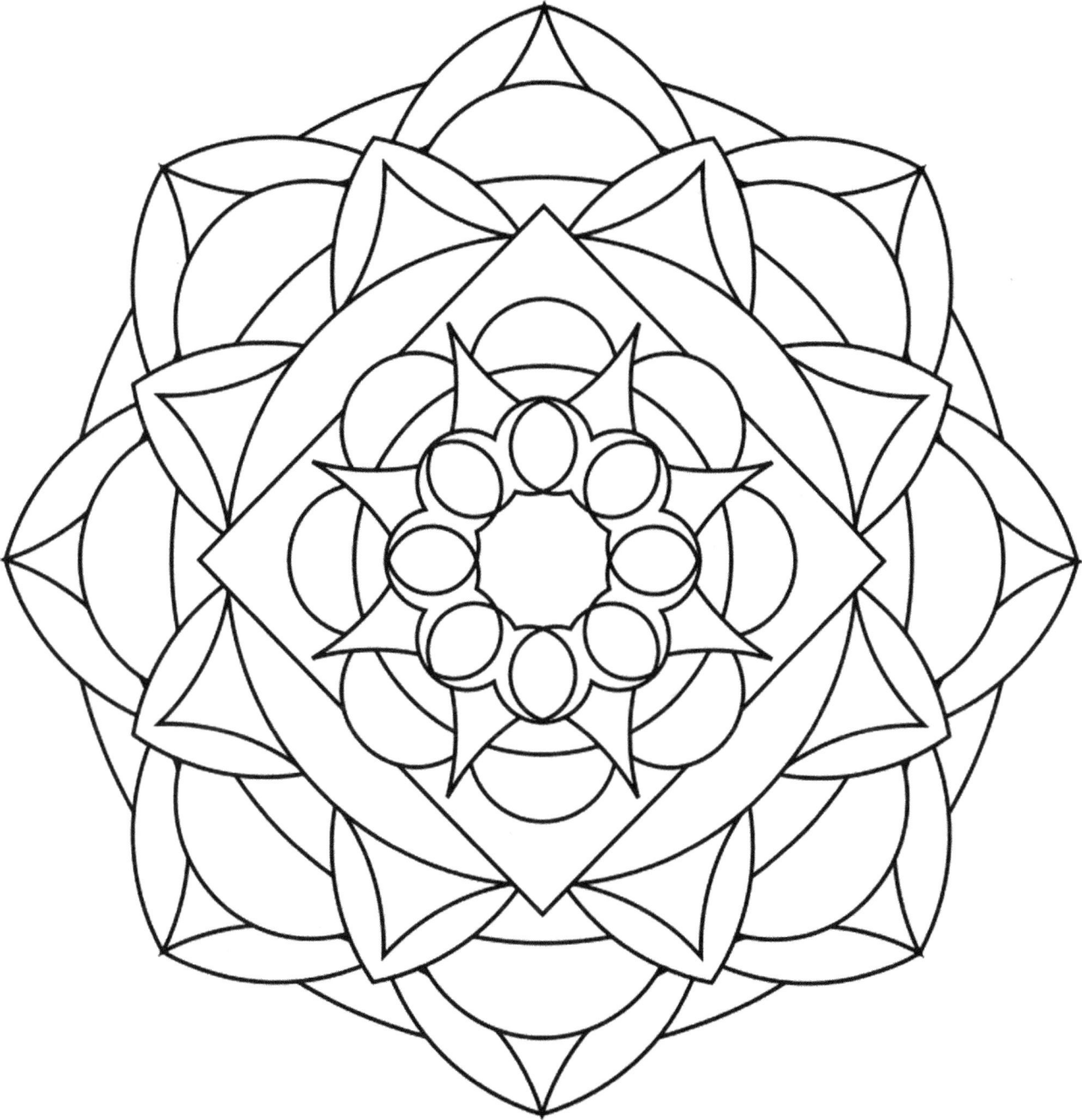

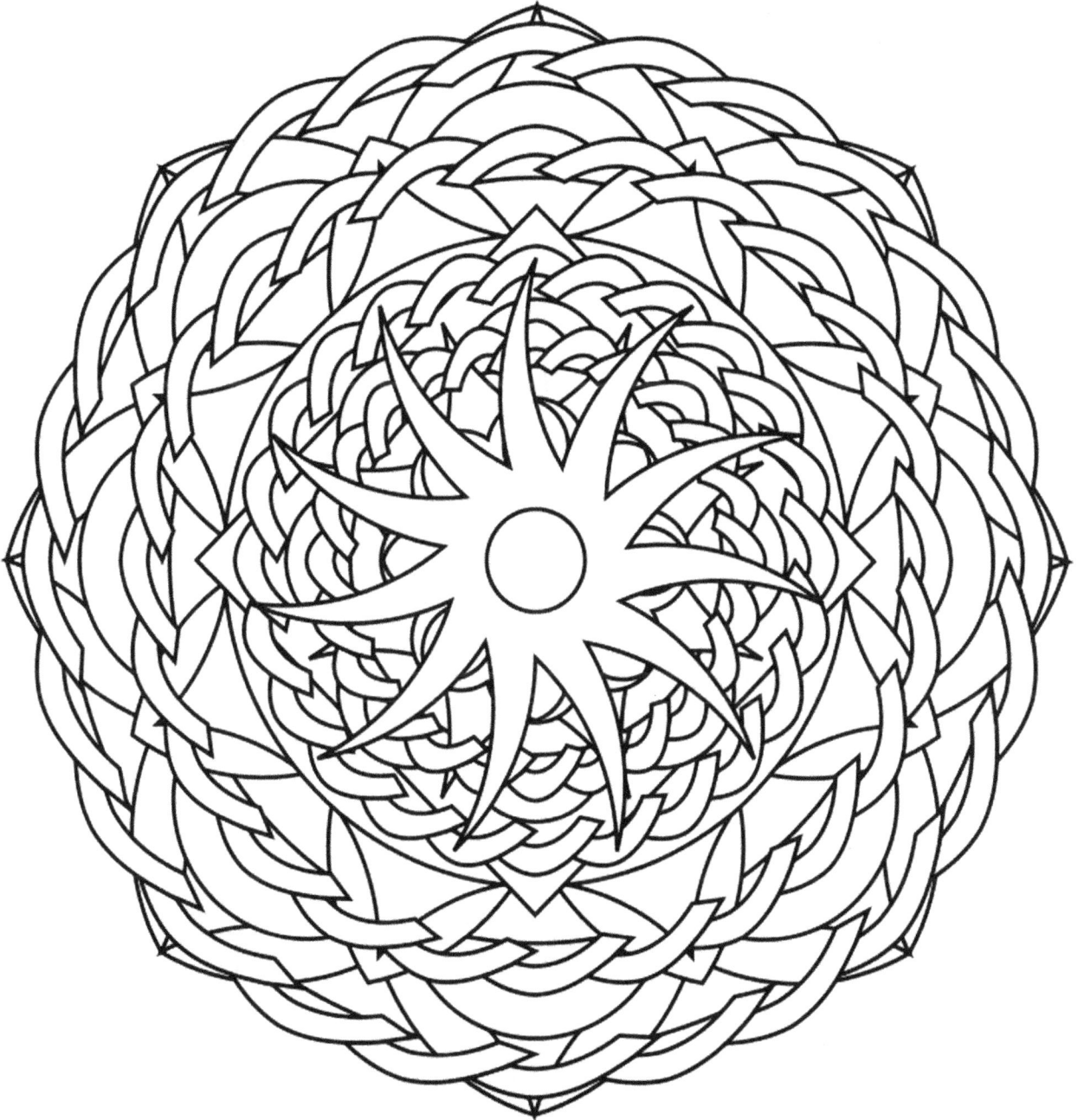

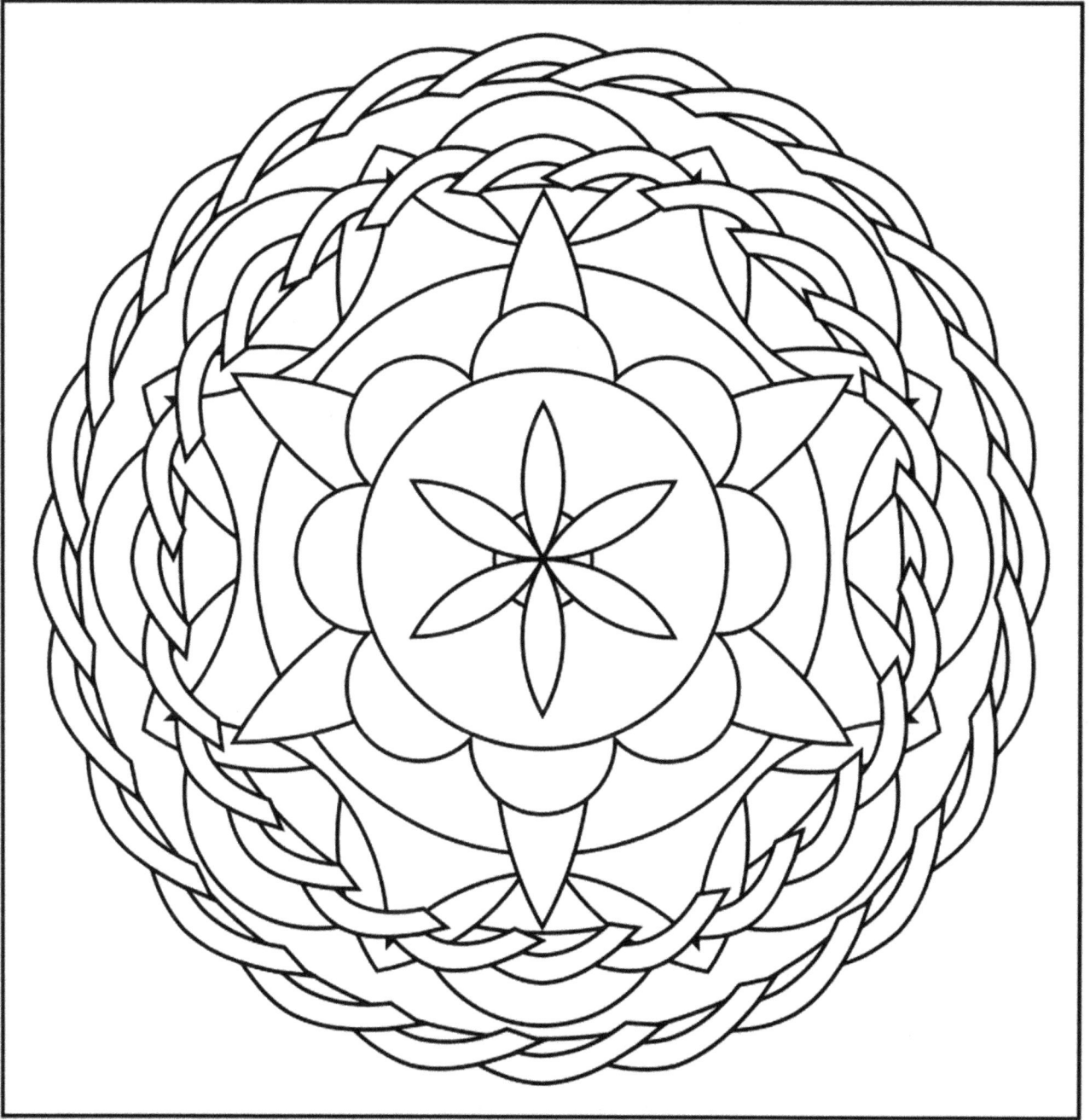

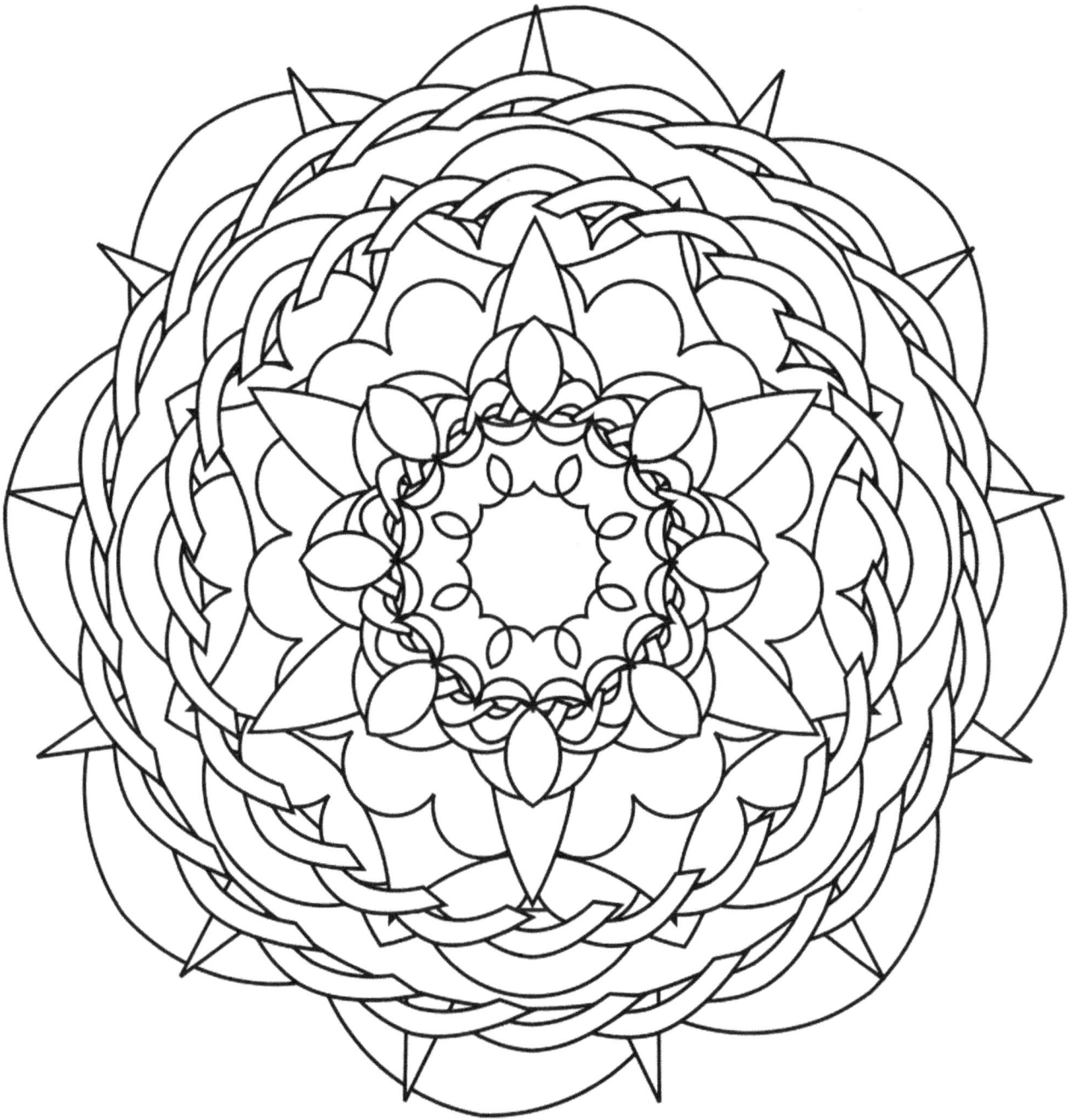

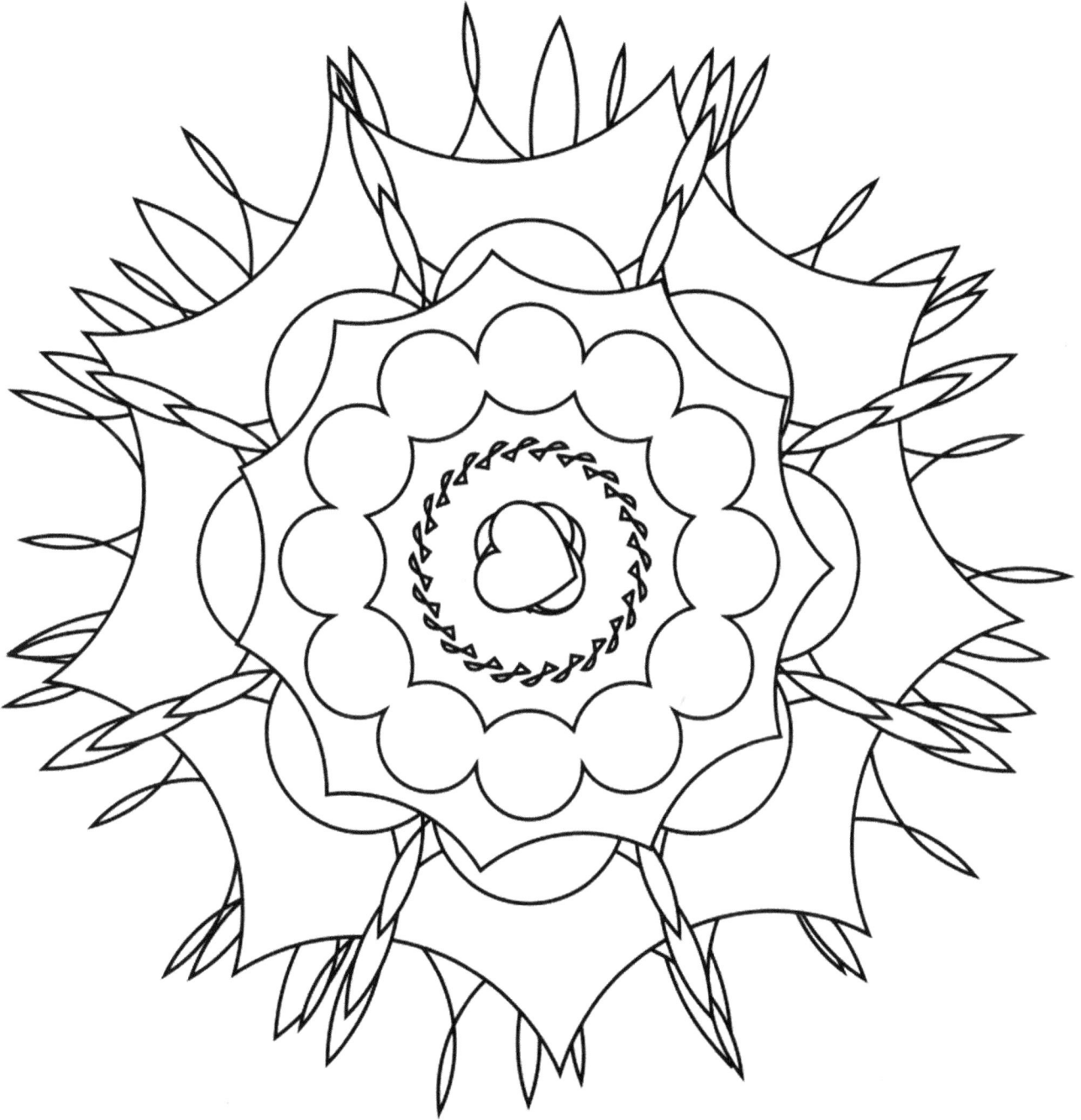

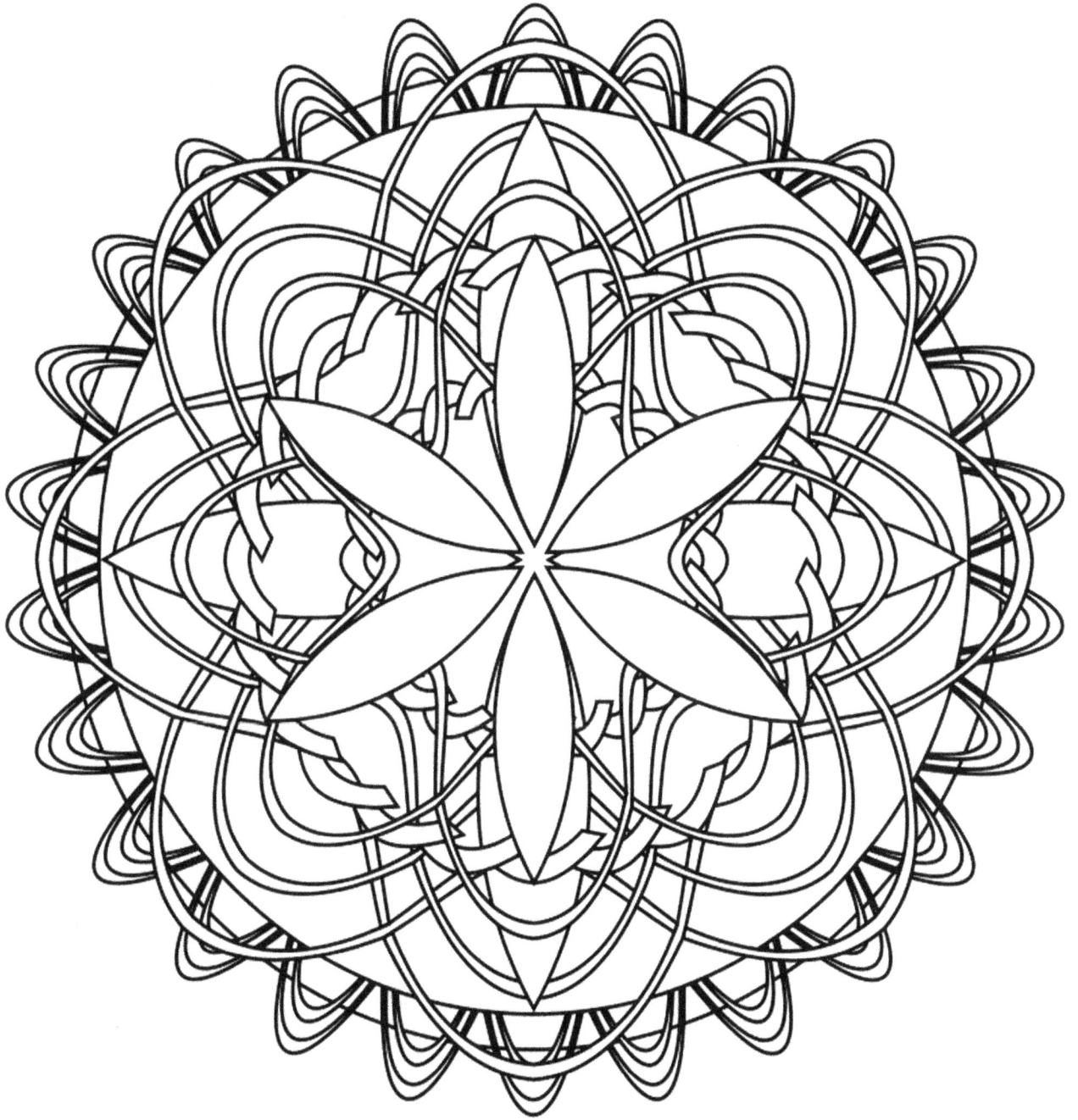

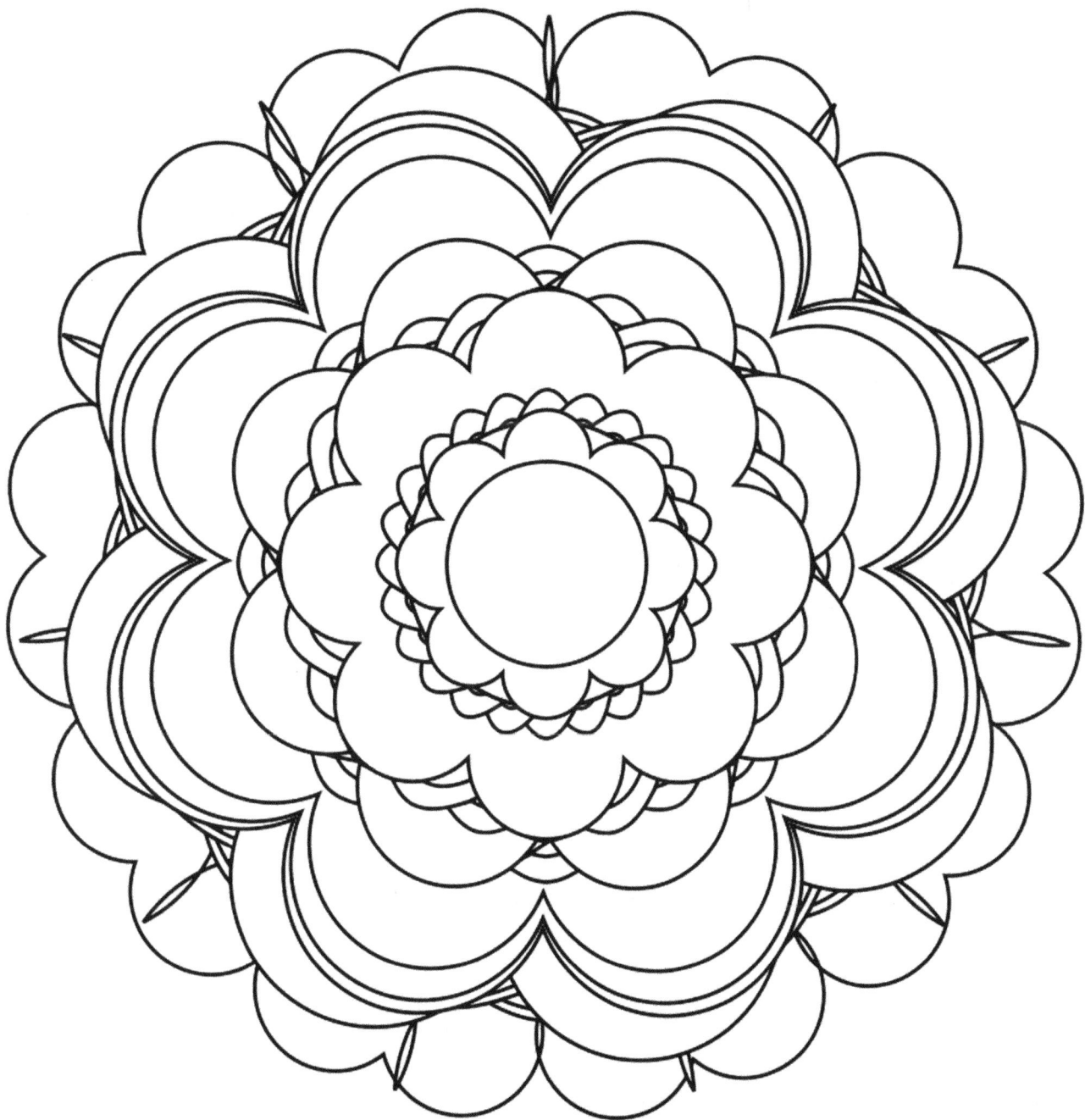

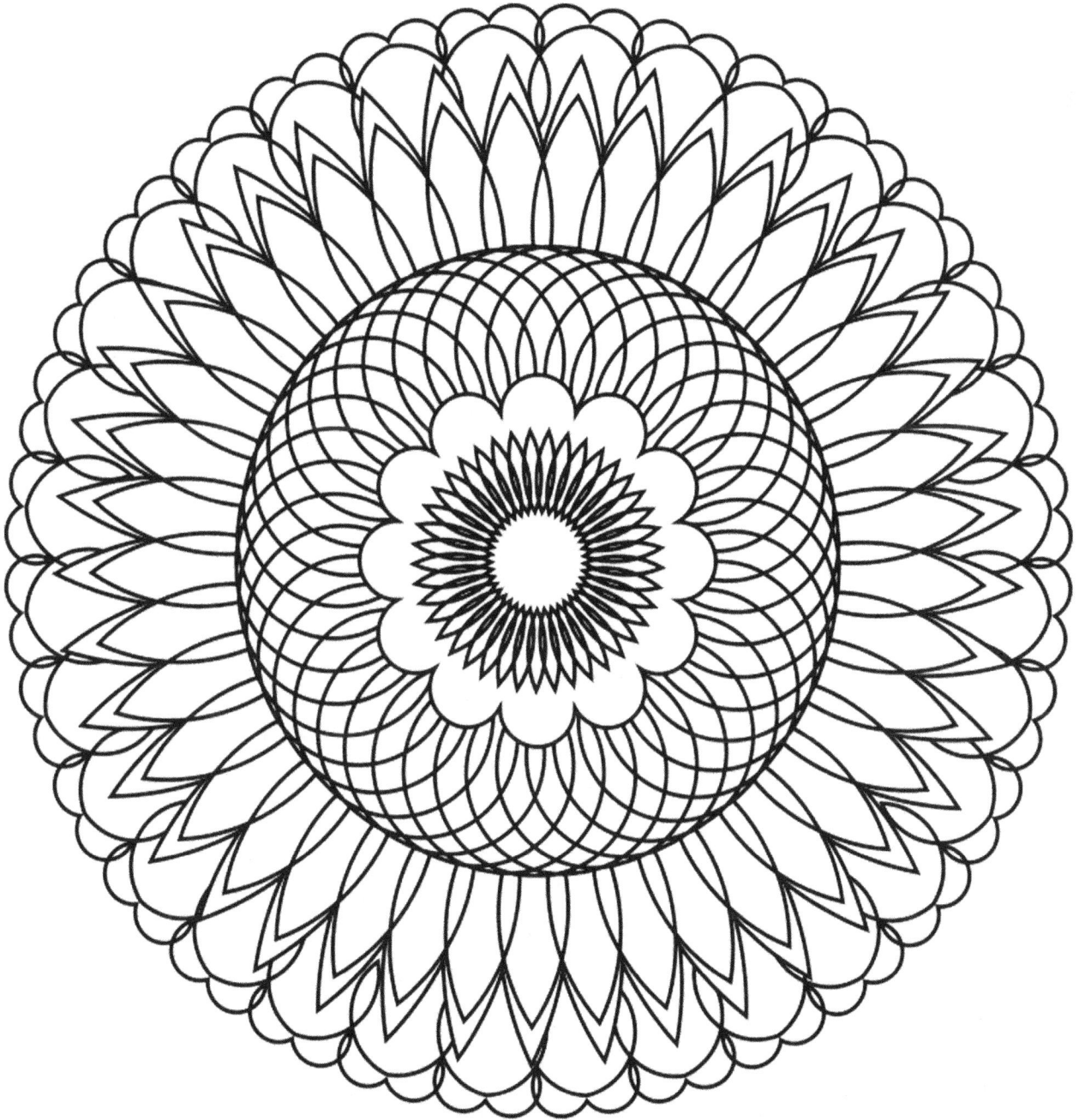

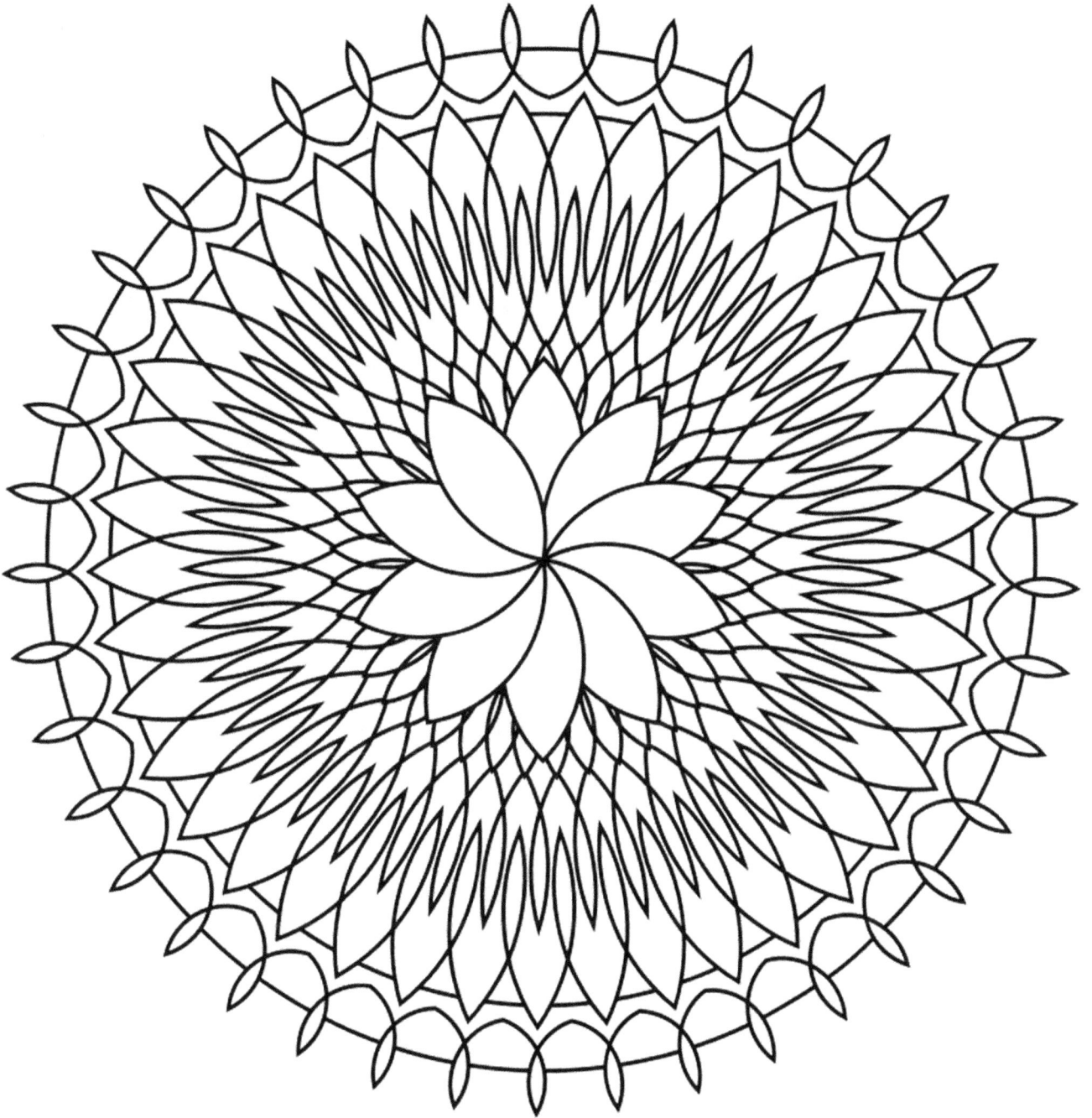

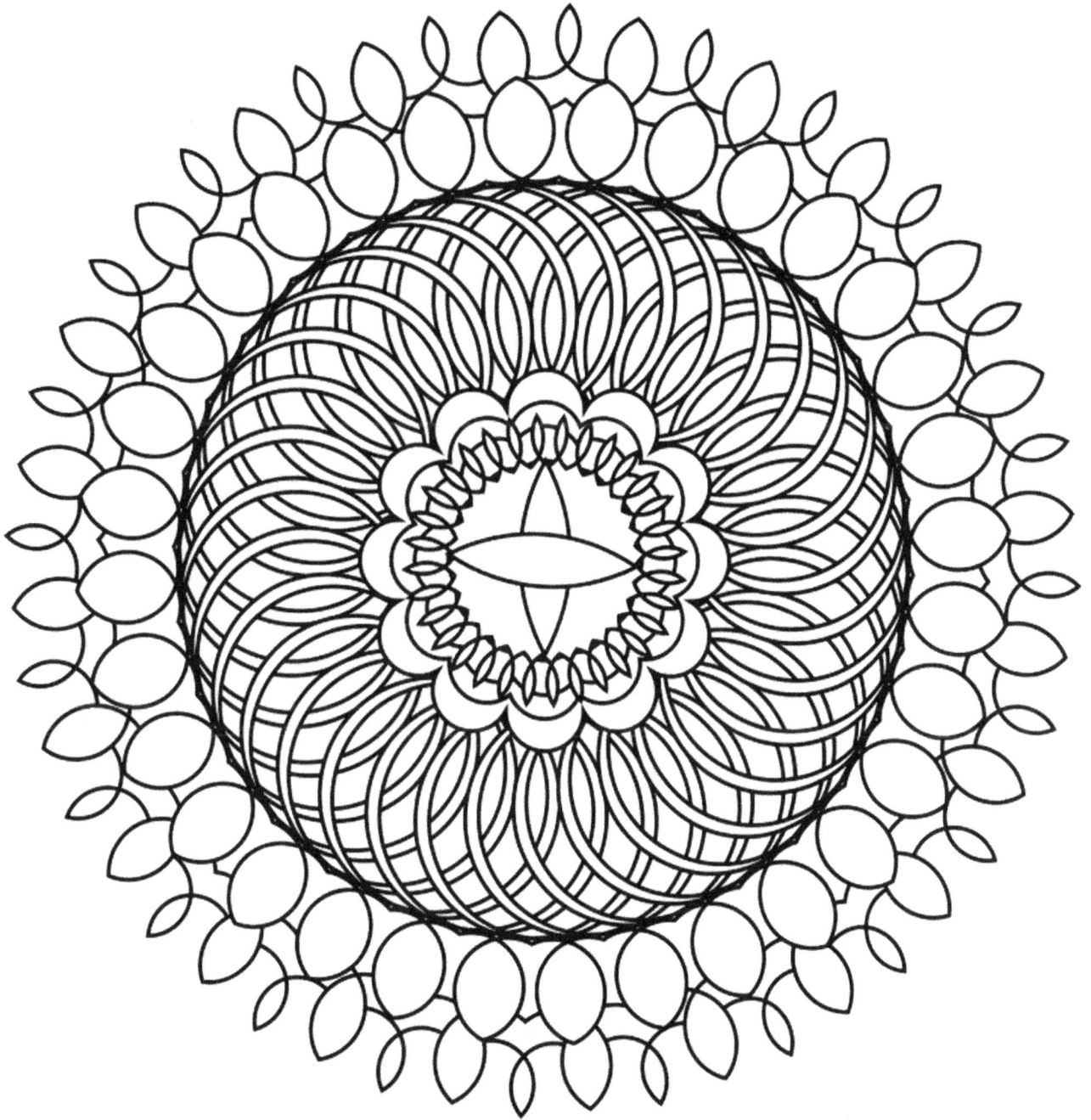

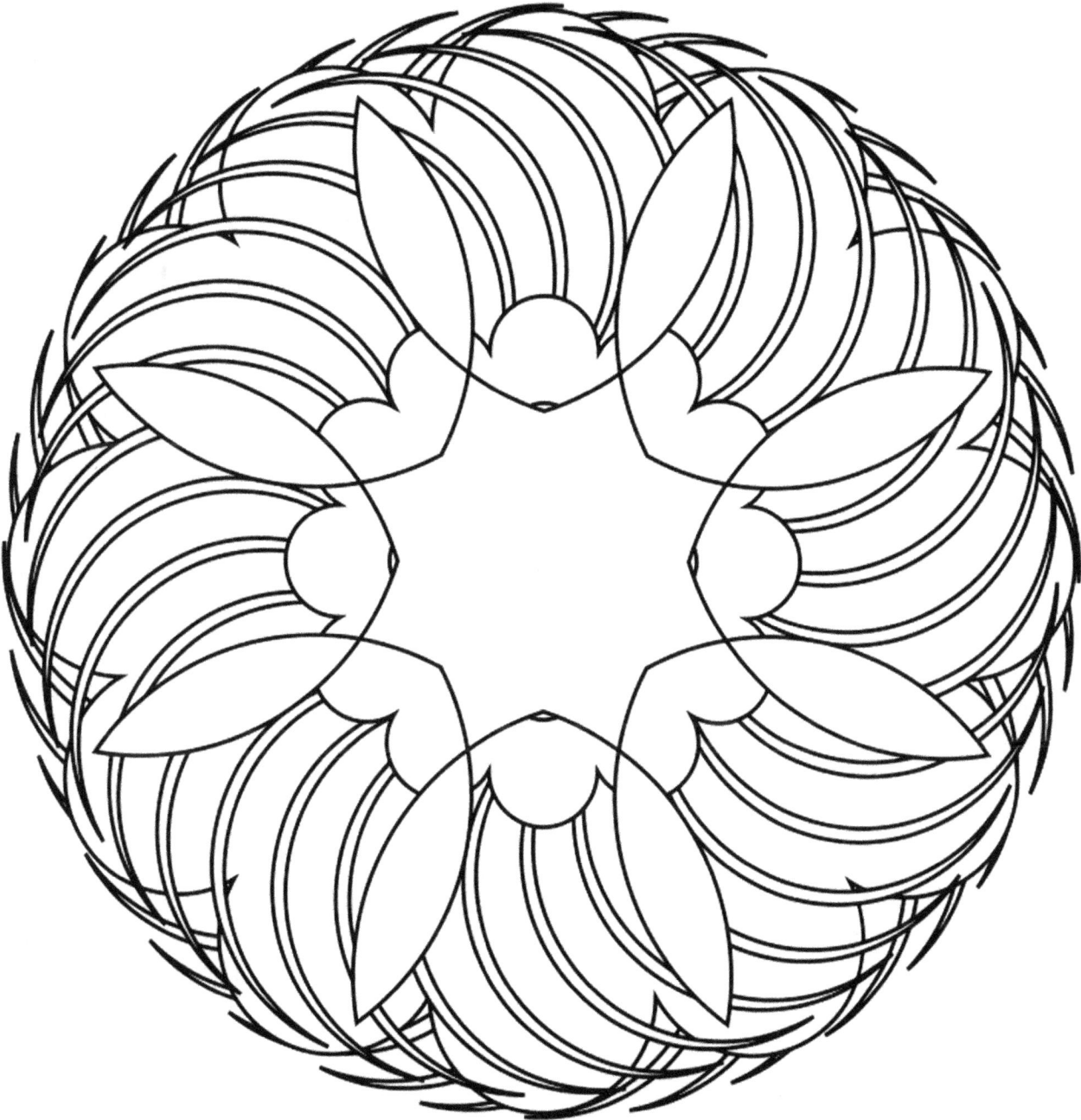

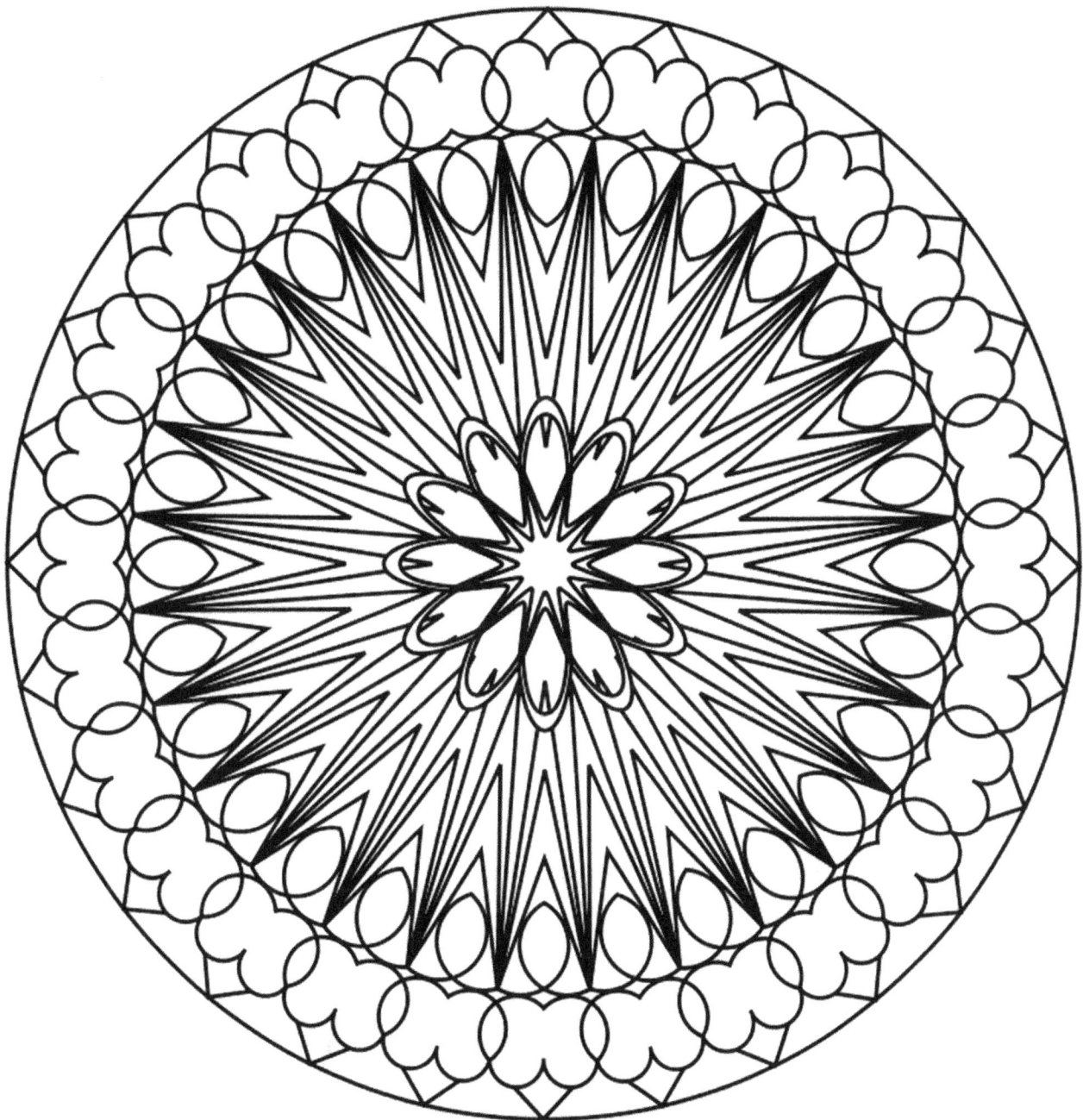

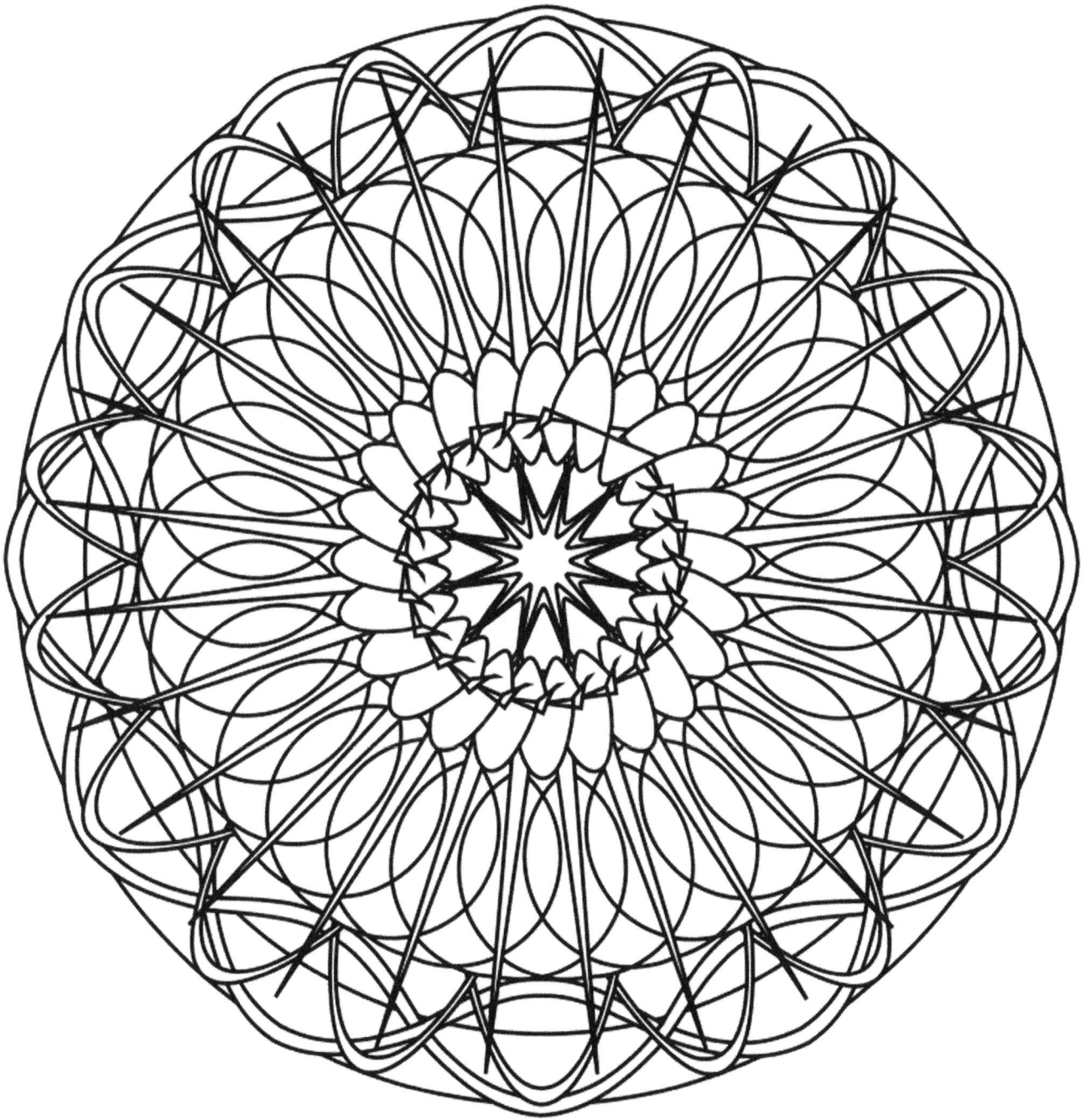

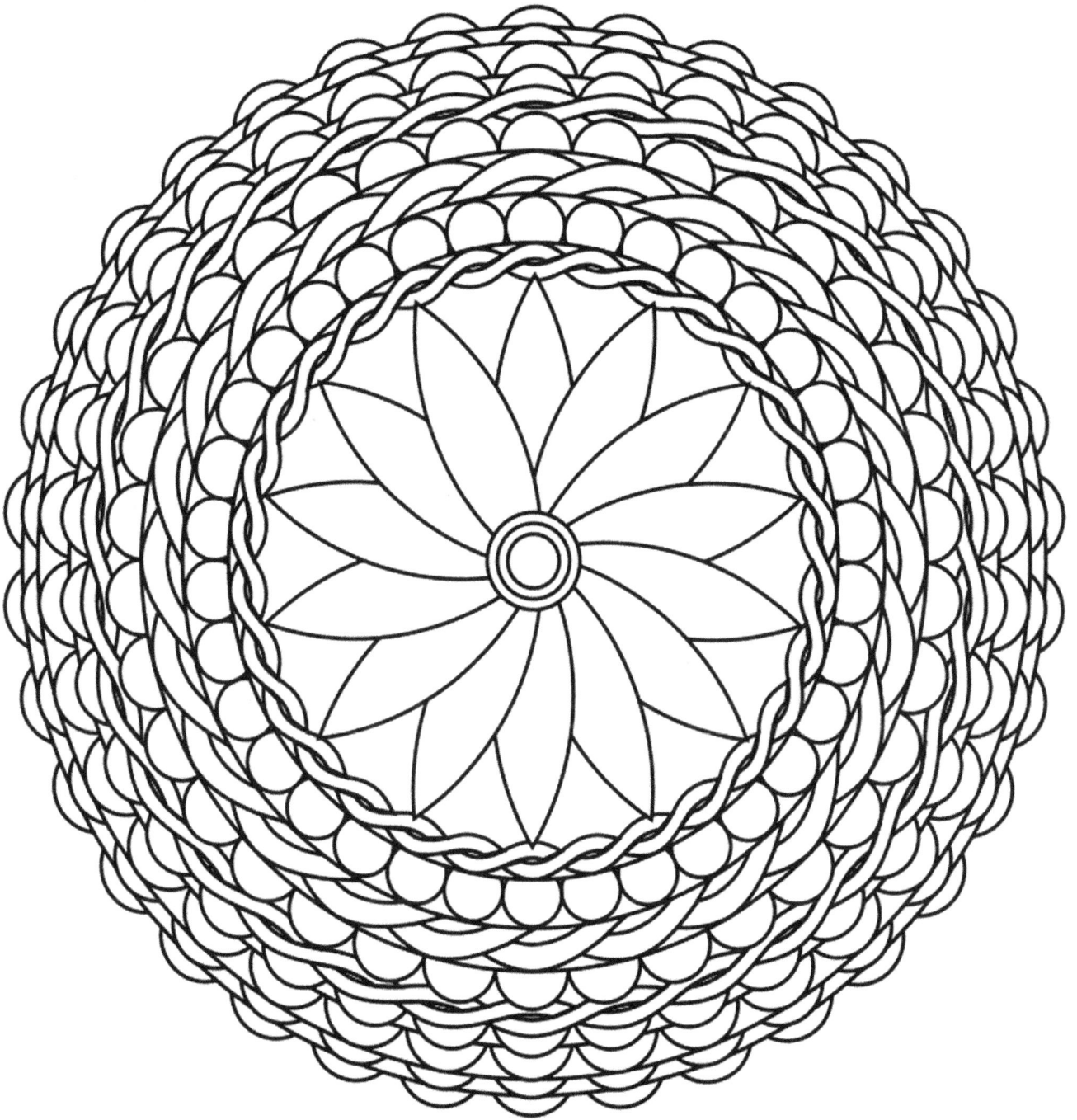

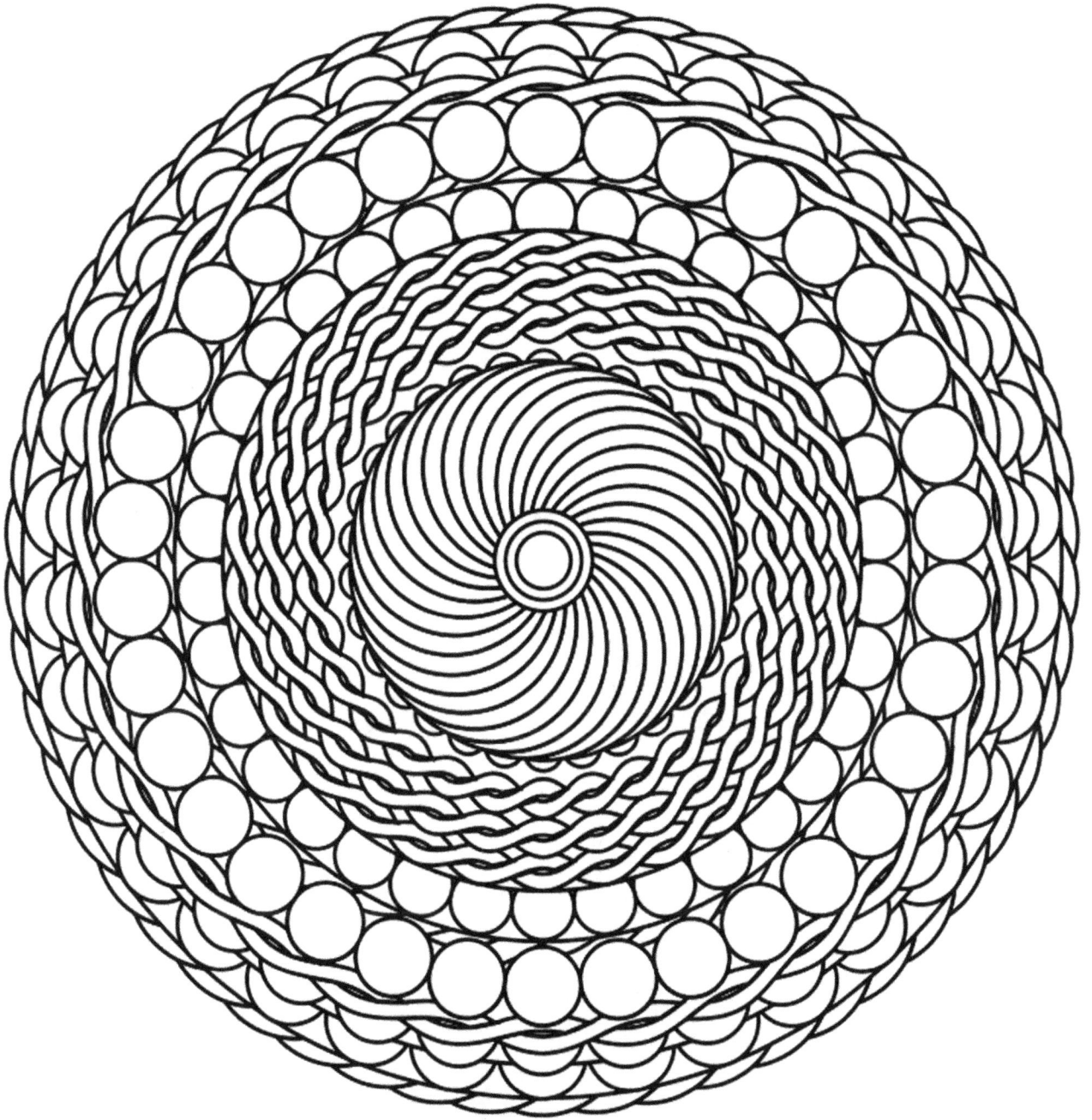

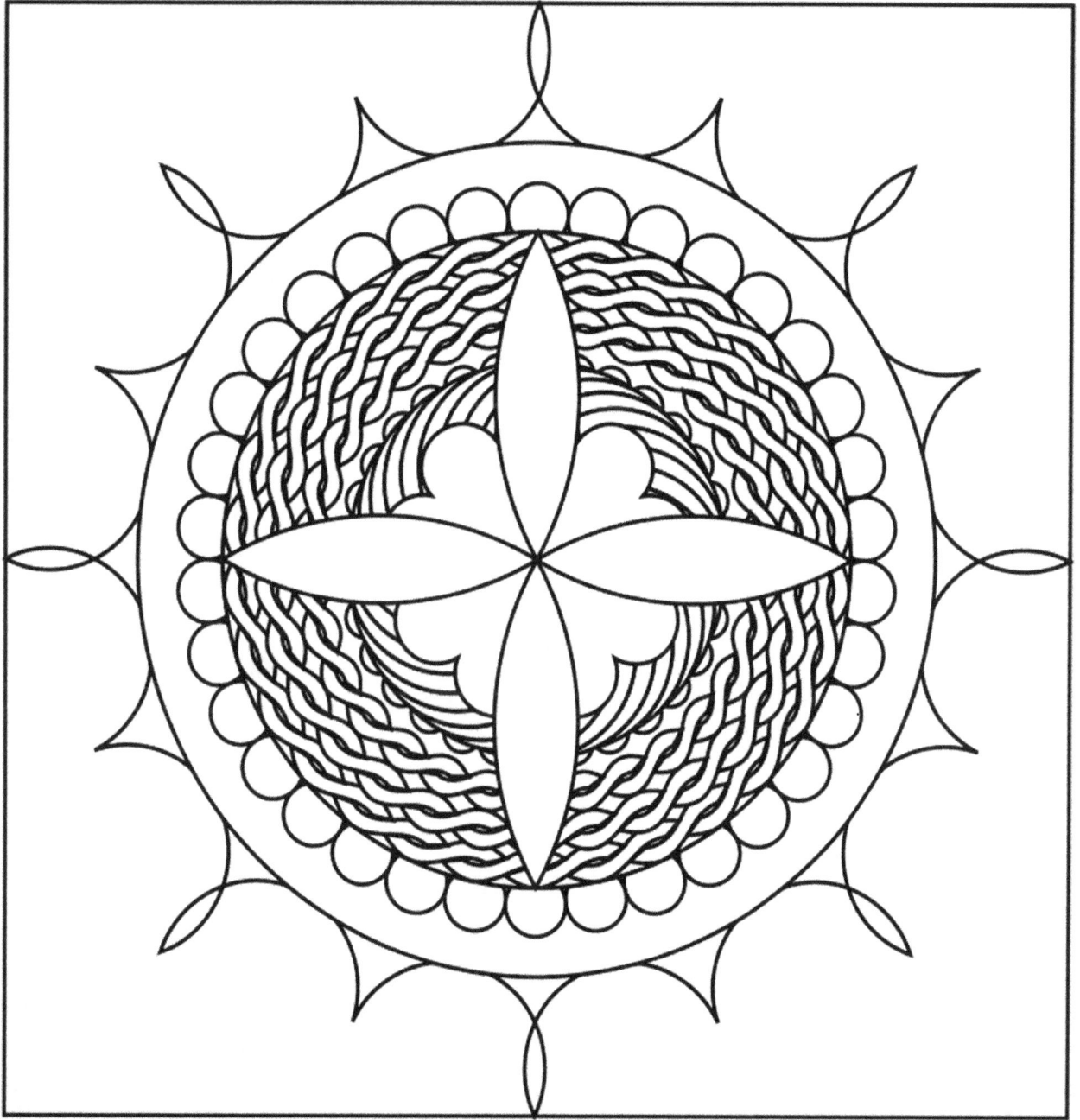

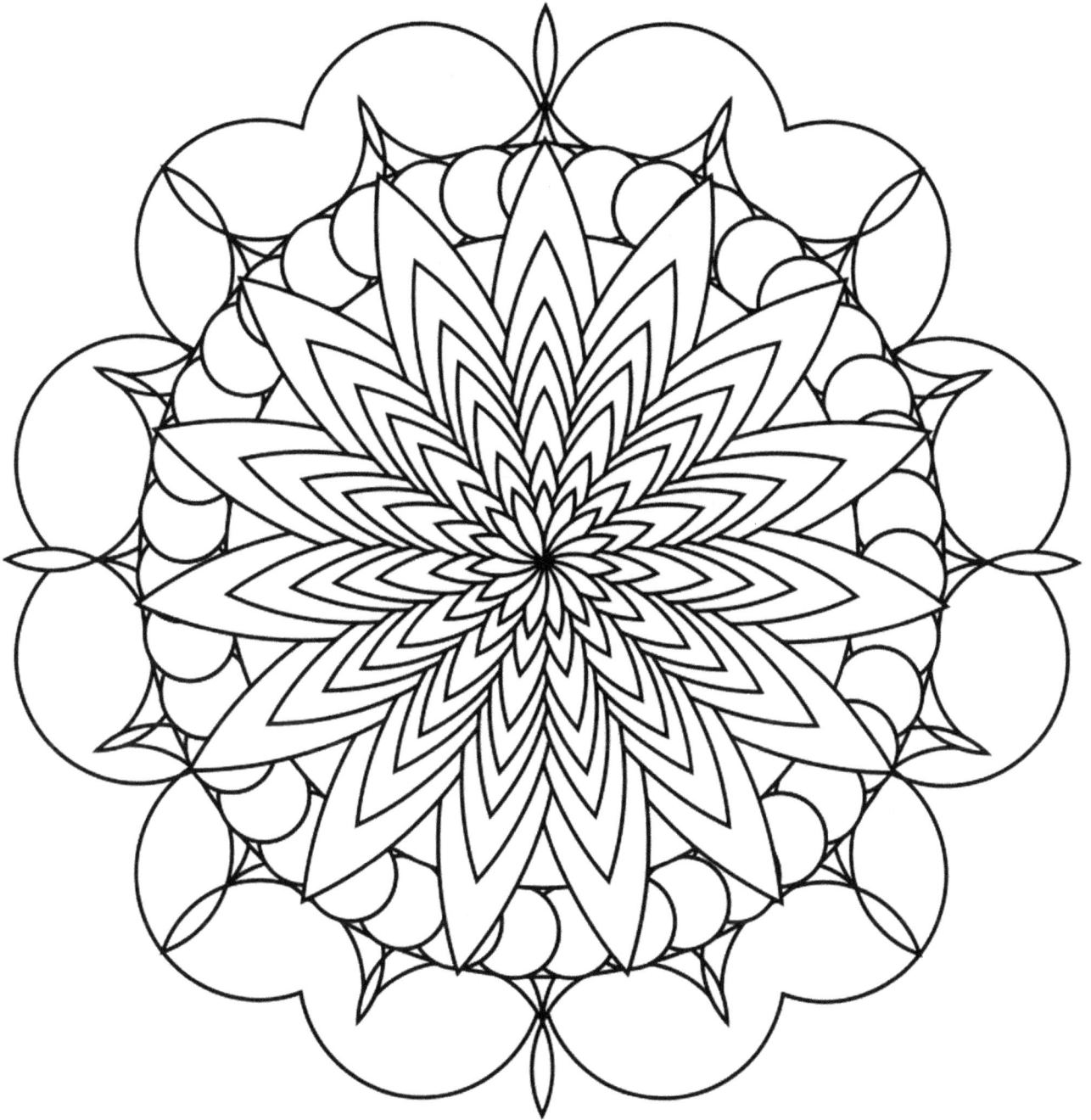

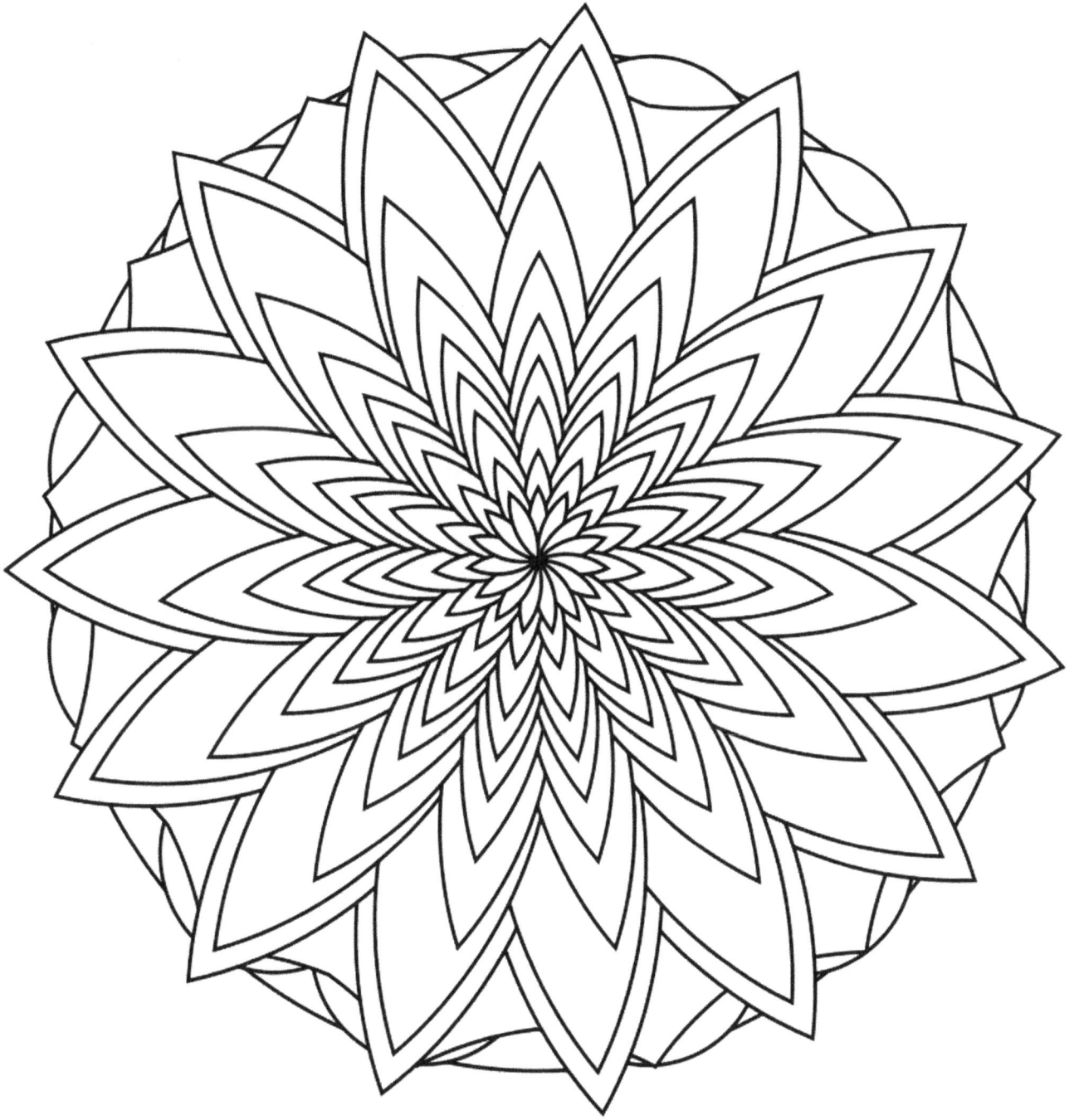

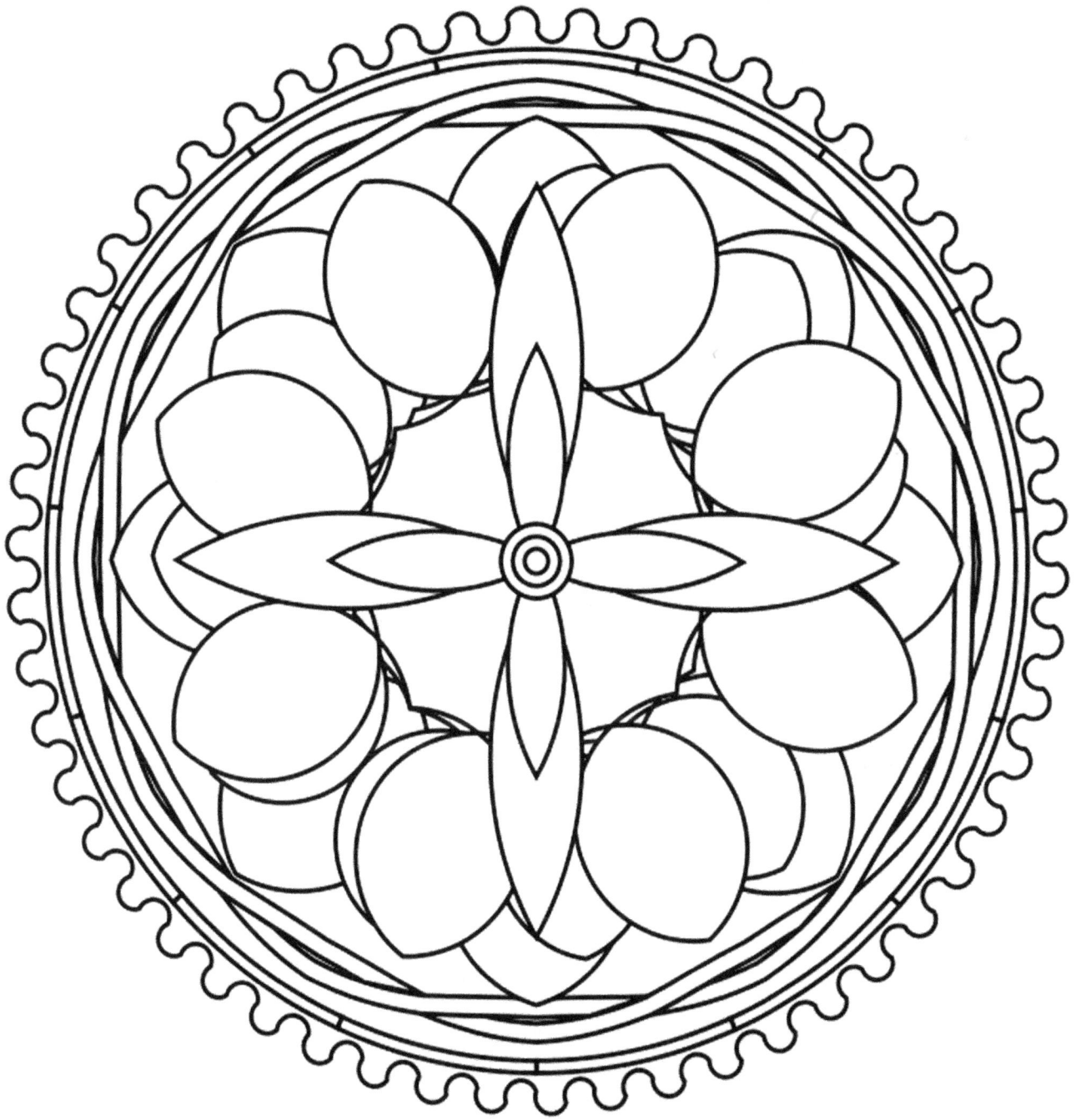

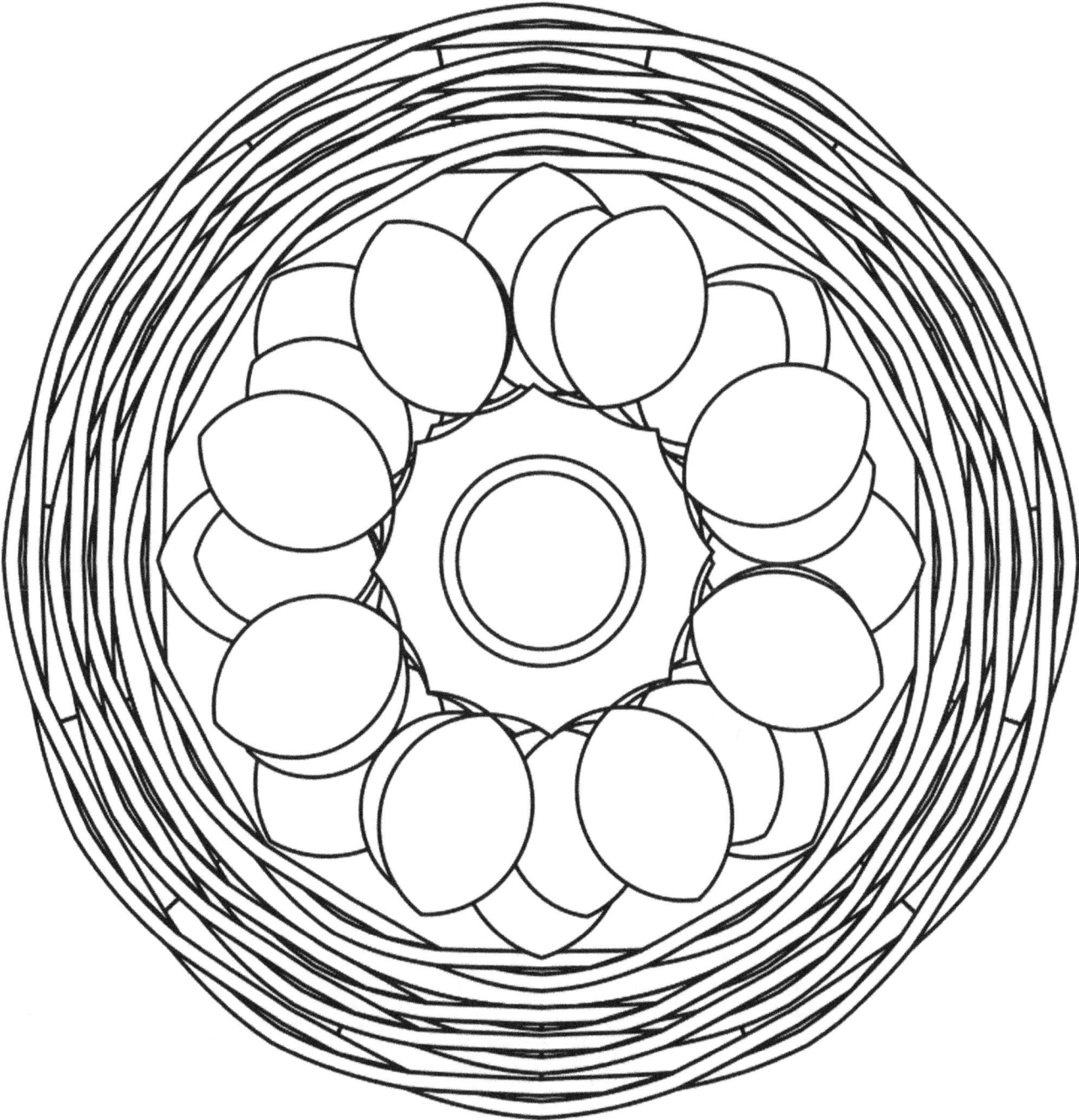

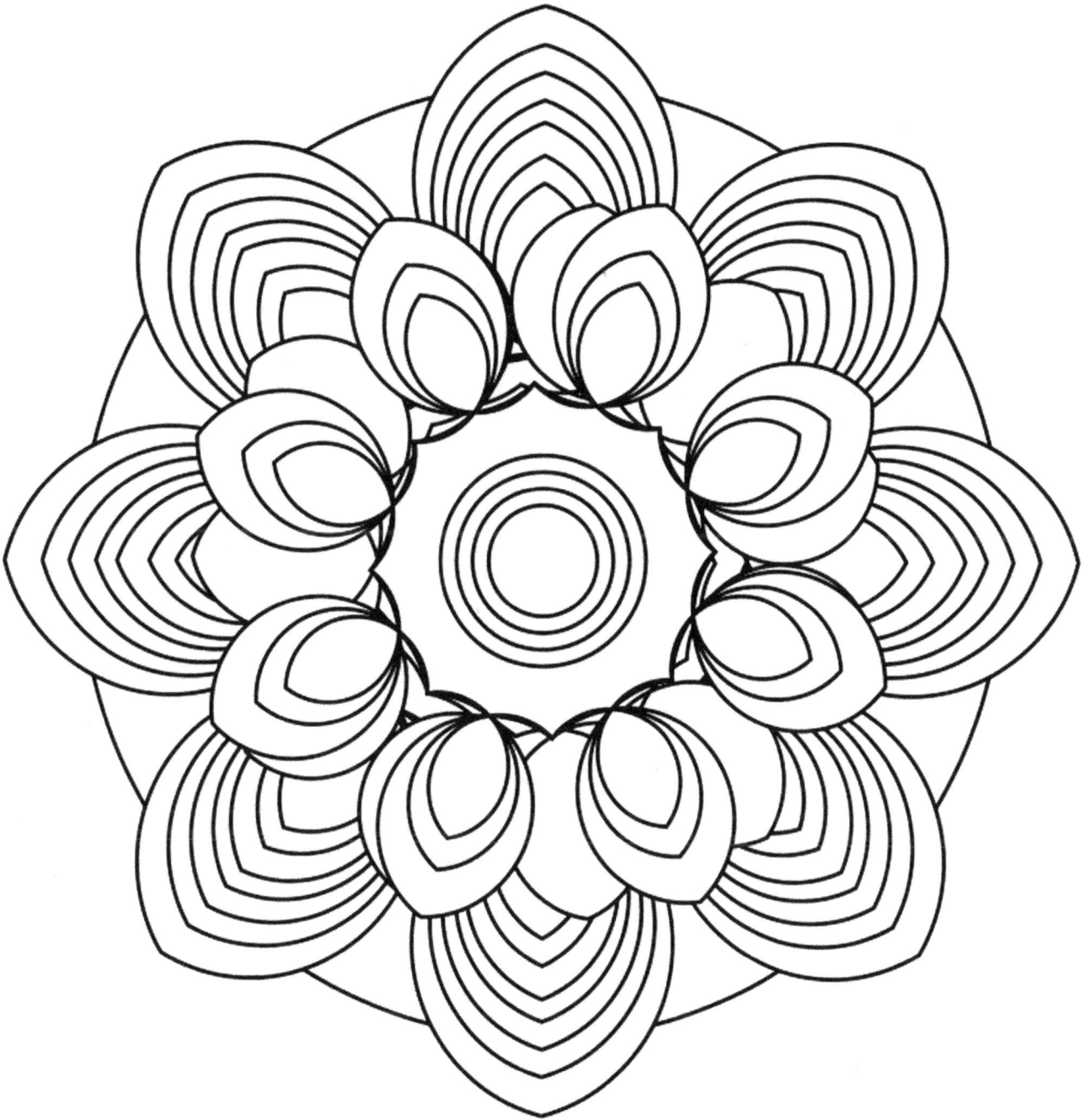

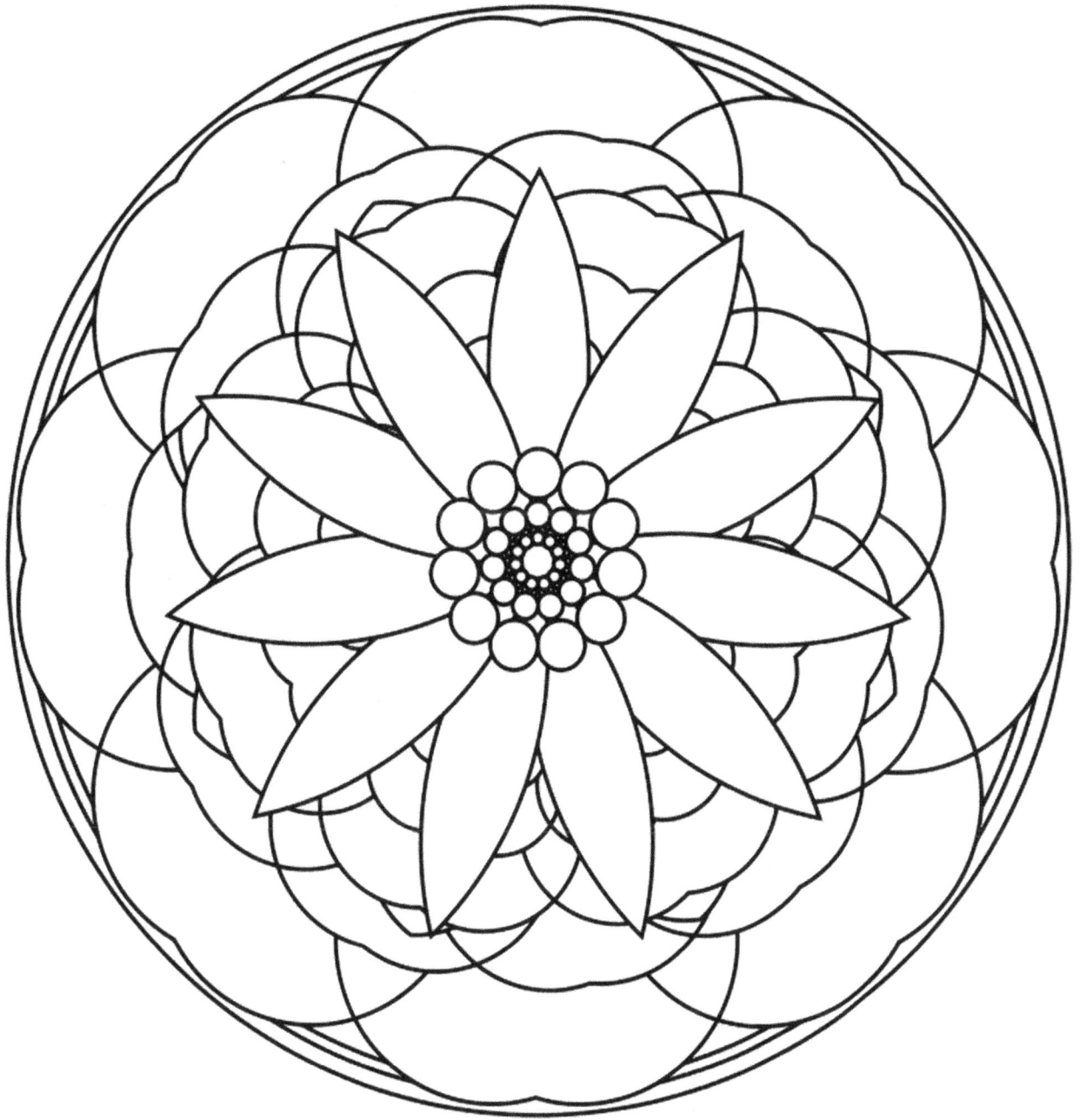

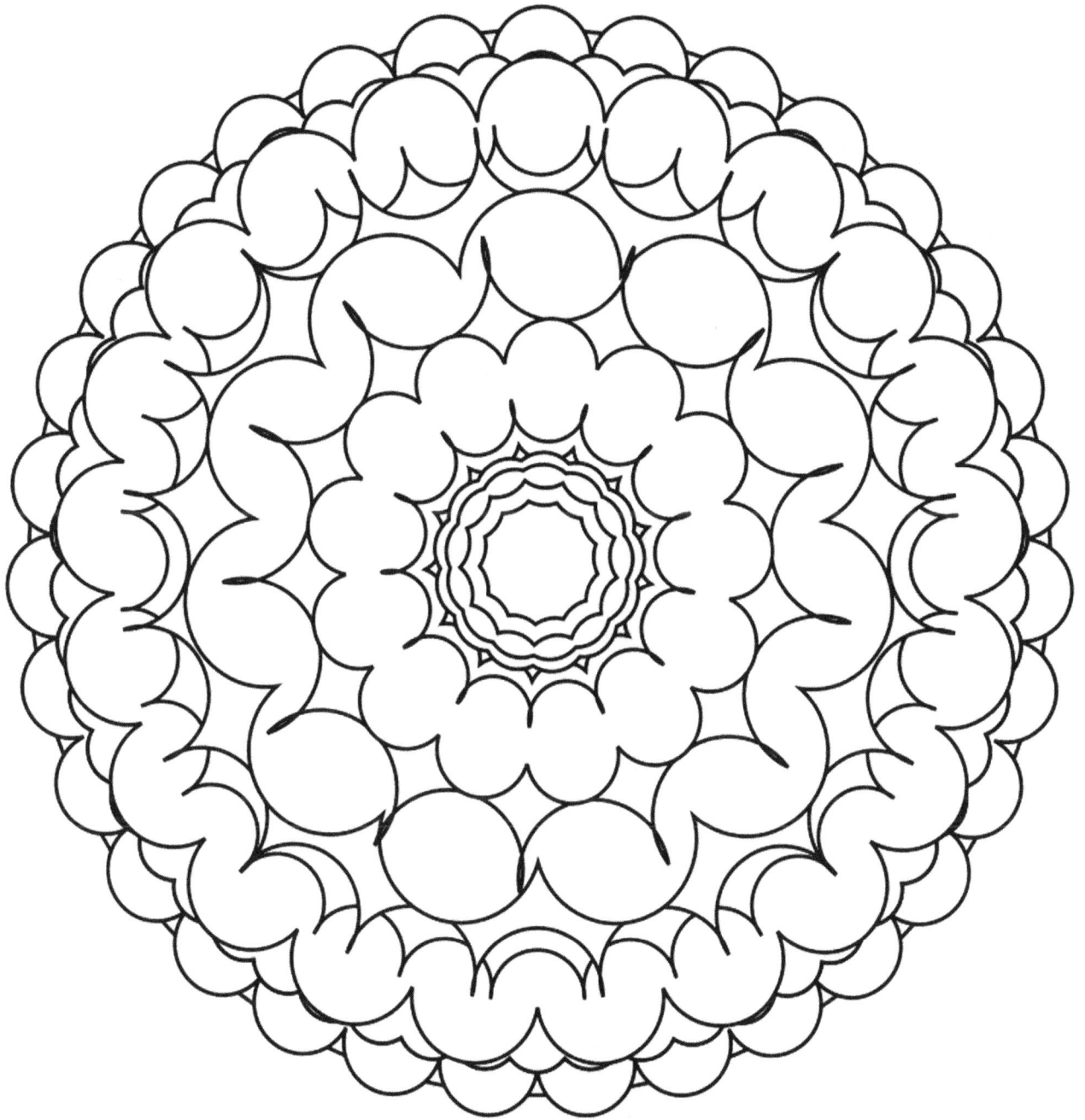

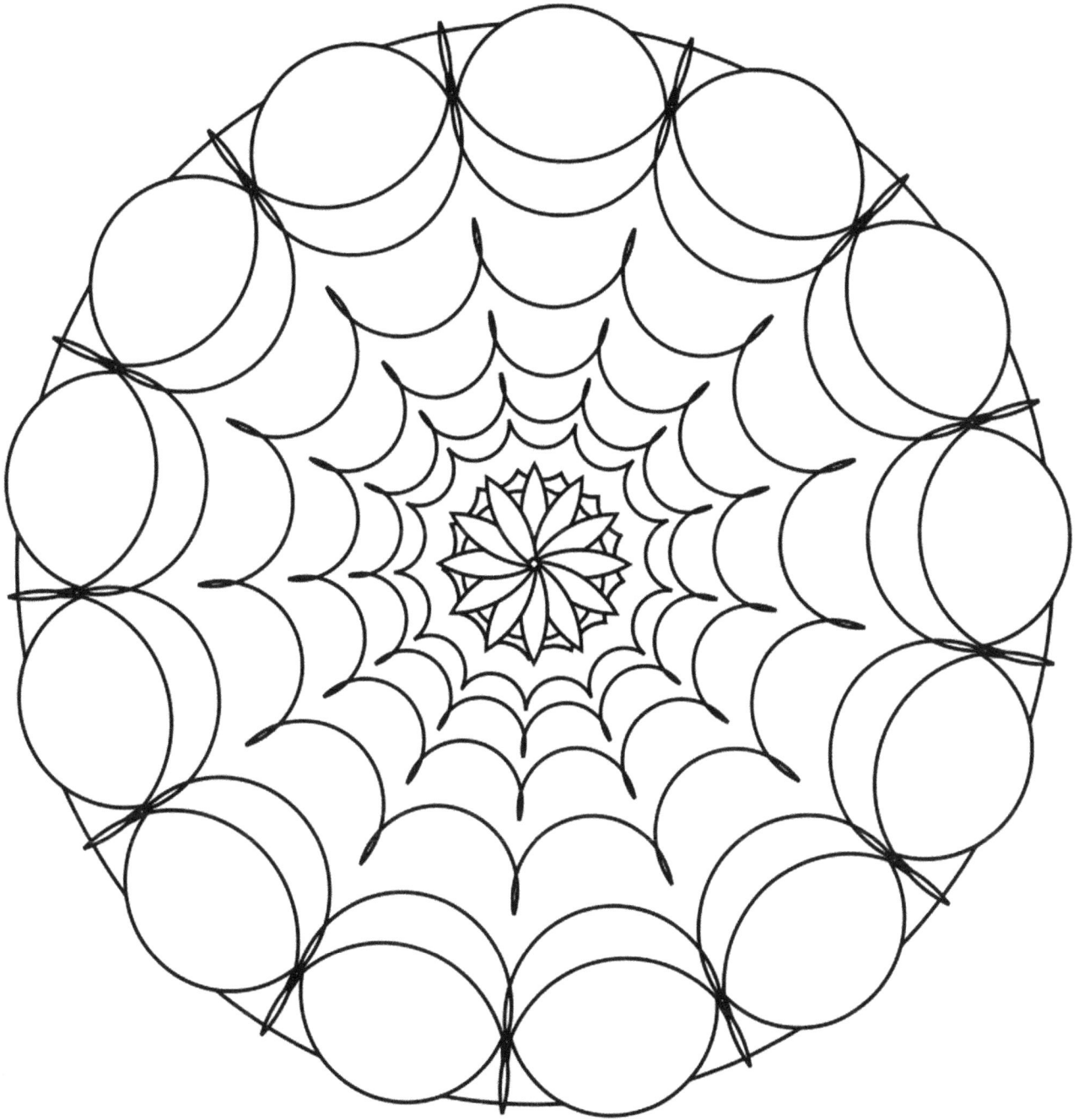

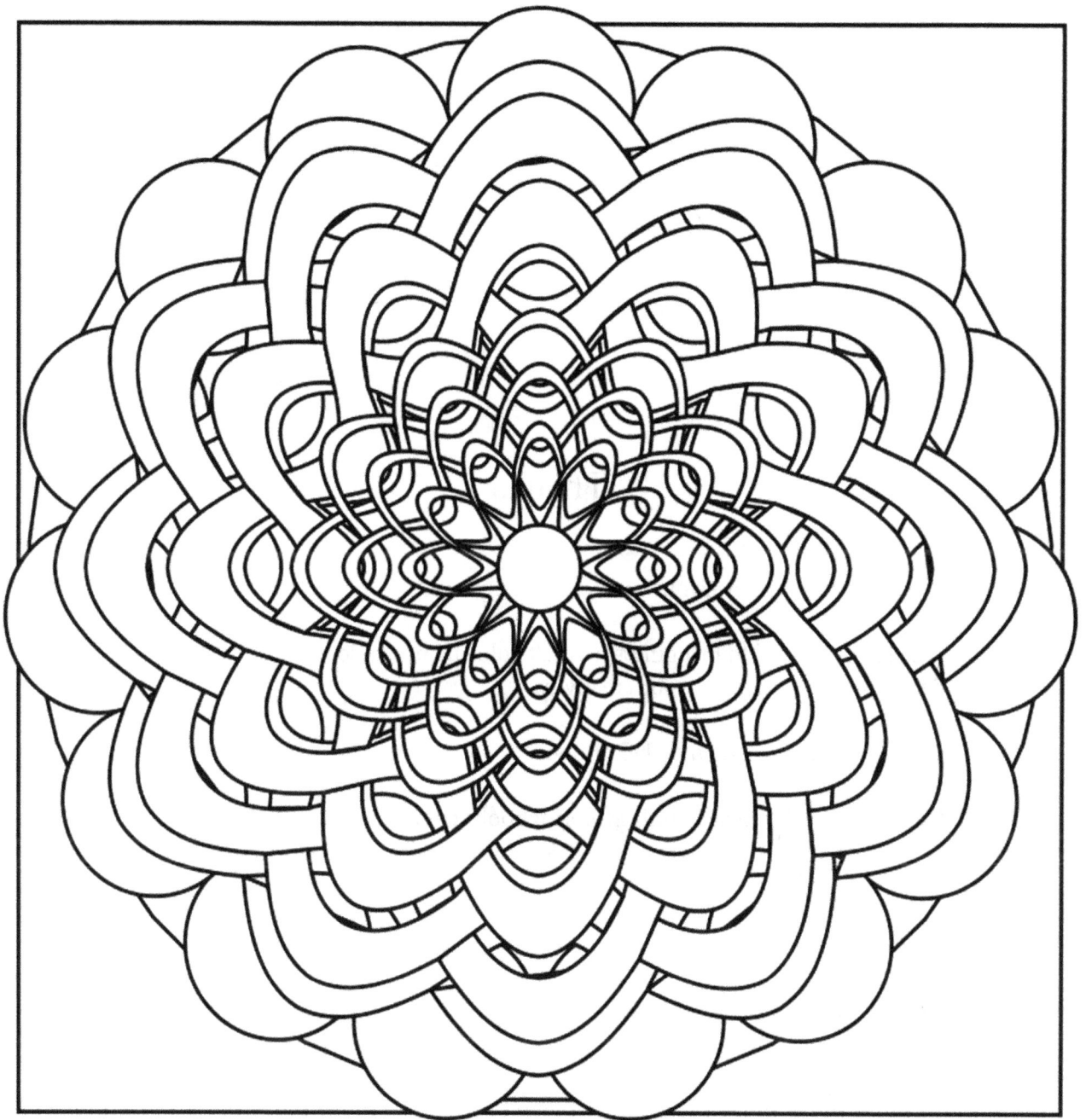

Thanks

A big thank you to everyone who colored my book.

We are committed to bringing you adult coloring books so you can relax, decompress and expand your creativity.

Concieved and designed by D.E. Boone.

Get the next edition at Calmingcoloringbooks.com

Dare To Be Calm

www.ingramcontent.com/pod-product-compliance
Lightning Source LLC
Chambersburg PA
CBHW081658270326
41933CB00017B/3209